ESSENTIALS OF
CLINICAL
NEUROANATOMY
and
NEUROPHYSIOLOGY

MANTER and GATZ'S

ESSENTIALS OF
CLINICAL
NEUROANATOMY
and
NEUROPHYSIOLOGY

RONALD G. CLARK, Ph.D.

Associate Professor
Department of Biological Structure
University of Miami School of Medicine

EDITION 5

F. A. DAVIS COMPANY, Philadelphia

Reprinted 1975

Library of Congress Cataloging in Publication Data

Manter, John Tinkham, 1910-
    Manter and Gatz's Essentials of clinical neuroanatomy and neurophysiology.

    First—4th ed. published under title: Essentials of clinical neuroanatomy and neurophysiology.
    Bibliography: p.
    1. Nervous system—Diseases.   2. Neurophysiology.
I. Gatz, Arthur John, 1907-   II. Clark, Ronald G.,
ed.   III. Title: Essentials of neuroanatomy and neurophysiology.   [DNLM: 1.   Nervous system—Anatomy and histology.   2. Neurophysiology.   WL100 M292e]
RC347.M32   1975   612'.8   74-10887
ISBN 0-8036-1850-6

Preface
to the fifth edition

While the basic objectives as set forth by the late Drs. Manter and Gatz are maintained, the present edition has undergone extensive revision.

A considerable portion of the information processed in the nervous system results in either facilitation or inhibition of muscular activity. Consequently, it is of the utmost importance that the student attains a good understanding of the pathways and structures associated with muscular tone and action. In this edition there is expanded coverage of the muscle spindle apparatus, cerebellum, basal ganglia, and all of the major areas of the central nervous system that exert an influence upon the descending pathways controlling motor cranial nerve nuclei and the anterior horn cells of the spinal cord.

The student will find it much easier to understand the intrinsic connections of the nervous system if he first studies the gross morphology of the brain and spinal cord, selected cross sections of which can then be examined in conjunction with the study of pathways as considered appropriate by the instructor. Several new figures concerning the anatomy of the nervous system have been added to the present edition. These, in addition to those already present in previous editions, enable the book to be used as an atlas in the laboratory.

The author expresses his deepest gratitude to Joe Witcher, Editor and Vice President of the F.A. Davis Company, for his continued support and counsel. Sincere thanks are also extended to Carol Levy and Marcia Athens for preparing the new illustrations.

RONALD G. CLARK

Preface
to the first edition

This book has been written with the object of providing a short, but comprehensive survey of the human nervous system. It is hoped that it will furnish a unified concept of structure and function which will be of practical value in leading to the understanding of the working mechanisms of the brain and spinal cord. Neither of these two aspects — structure and function — stands apart from the other. Together they furnish the key to the significance of the abnormal changes in function that go hand in hand with structural lesions of the nervous system. The viewpoints of three closely dependent sciences — neuroanatomy, neurophysiology and clinical neurology — are combined and used freely, not with the intent of covering these fields exhaustively, but in the belief that a more discerning approach to the study of the nervous system can be attained by bringing together all three facets of the subject.

To suit the needs of the medical student, or the physician who wishes to review the nervous system efficiently, basic information is presented in concise form. Consequently, it has not been feasible to cite published reports of research from which present concepts of the nervous system have evolved. The planning and arrangement of the chapters are such that whole topics can be covered rapidly. Presenting the subject material to classes in this form allows more time for discussion and review, or, if the teacher desires, for lectures dealing with advanced aspects, than would otherwise be permitted.

For the encouragement and valuable suggestions they have given me, I am indebted to my former colleague, Dr. William H. Waller, Jr., and to Dr. Lester L. Bowles. I am deeply grateful to Mr. A. H. Germagian for executing most of the drawings and diagrams, and to Mr. Richard Meyers for his special assistance with the illustrations.

JOHN T. MANTER

Contents

1   Introduction   1
2   Functional Components of the Spinal Nerves   10
3   Spinal Reflexes and Muscle Tone   13
4   The Descending Motor Pathways   18
5   The Anterolateral System   24
6   Proprioception and Stereognosis   31
7   Tactile Senses   36
8   Lesions of Nerves and Spinal Cord   40
9   Brain Stem   50
10 Functional Components of the Cranial Nerves   63
11 Cranial Nerves of the Medulla   70
12 Cranial Nerves of the Pons and Midbrain   79
13 Hearing   86
14 The Vestibular System   91
15 The Cerebellum   97
16 Lesions of the Brain Stem   105
17 Vision   112
18 Optic Reflexes   116
19 The Autonomic Nervous System   120
20 The Hypothalamus and Limbic System   127
21 The Thalamus   134
22 Rhinencephalon and Olfactory Reflexes   141
23 The Cerebral Cortex   145
24 The Basal Ganglia and Related Structures   160
25 The Cerebrospinal Fluid   167
Index   172

1
Introduction

Nerve Cells and Nerve Fibers

The *neuron* (nerve cell) is the functional and anatomical unit of the nervous system. Each consists of a *cell body* (perikaryon) and one to several dozen processes of varying length called nerve fibers. *Dendrites* are short branching fibers which receive impulses and conduct them *toward* the nerve cell body. The term *axon*, in a strict sense, applies to a single long fiber that conducts impulses *away* from a nerve cell body. Any long fiber, however, is commonly referred to as an axon regardless of the direction of conduction.

Nerve cell bodies are usually located in groups. Outside of the brain and spinal cord such groups are called *ganglia*. In the cortex of the cerebrum and cerebellum, nerve cells are arranged in very extensive laminated sheets. Elsewhere within the brain and spinal cord they form groups of various sizes and shapes known as *nuclei*. In this instance the term nucleus has a different meaning from the nucleus of an individual cell. Those regions of the brain and spinal cord that contain aggregations of nerve cell bodies comprise the *gray matter* and, in the fresh state, they are grayish in color. The remaining areas consist primarily of myelinated nerve fibers and make up the *white matter*.

Some nerve fibers are naked axis cylinders, but most of them are encased in a sheath. Many of the peripheral nerve fibers have a myelin sheath and a neurolemma (sheath of Schwann) as well. Actually, both sheaths are the products of Schwann cells and thus are inseparable. Peripheral autonomic fibers (postganglionic) have no

1

myelin sheath but retain a neurolemma. The myelinated fibers that are located in the white matter of the brain and spinal cord possess a myelin sheath but have no neurolemma. Small, circumferential gaps, *nodes of Ranvier*, occur periodically in the myelin sheath. That portion of the myelinated axon between the nodes is called the internode. Action potentials, produced when the spike region of a neuron is sufficiently depolarized by the action of presynaptic neurotransmitters, travel by jumping from node to node. This process is referred to as *saltatory conduction* and it is responsible for causing successive depolarizations.

Nerve fibers of the brain and spinal cord that have a common origin and a common destination constitute a tract. Although a tract occupies a regular position, it does not always form a compact bundle because of some dispersion with intermingling fibers of neighboring tracts. There are a number of bundles of fibers in the brain that are so distinct anatomically that they have been given the names *fasciculus, brachium, peduncle, column,* or *lemniscus.* These may contain only a single tract or they may comprise several running together in the same bundle. Nerve, nerve root, nerve trunk, nerve cord, and ramus are appropriate anatomical terms for bundles of nerve fibers outside the brain and spinal cord.

Transmission of impulses from neuron to neuron occurs at a synapse—a place where fine branches of one neuron are in contact with the cell body or processes of another neuron. Action potentials in the *presynaptic* neuron cause the release of *neurotransmitters* from *synaptic vesicles* which traverse the *synaptic cleft* and either prevent or produce action potentials in the *postsynaptic* neuron. Synaptic ramifications of dendrites and terminal branches of axons form a delicate network throughout the gray substance known as *neuropile.* Nerve cells are normally stimulated at only one set of terminals and thus conduct impulses in only one direction—away from the region which receives stimulation. *Afferent fibers* (dendrites) conduct the impulse toward the cell body; *efferent fibers* conduct away from the cell body. The fibers of the dorsal roots of the spinal cord, for example, are spinal afferents. It is customary to name fibers by formulating a compound word which contains the name of their place of origin followed by the name of their termination. For example, thalamocortical fibers go from the thalamus to the cerebral cortex.

The Peripheral Nervous System

The cranial and spinal nerves with their associated ganglia make up the peripheral nervous system. Motor fibers of peripheral nerves are of two types: *somatic motor fibers* which terminate in *skeletal muscle,* and *autonomic fibers* which innervate *cardiac muscle, smooth muscle,* and *glands.* The sensory fibers of nerves transmit signals from receptor end organs of various types. Each fiber conducts impulses toward the spinal cord and brain from the particular receptor with which it is connected.

The Central Nervous System

The central nervous system (CNS) consists of the brain and the spinal cord. The brain of the young adult male averages 1380 gm in weight (generally 100 gm less in females). The brain is divided into three gross parts, the cerebrum, the brain stem, and the cerebellum.

The Cerebrum

The two cerebral hemispheres are incompletely separated by a deep, *medial longitudinal fissure.* They are joined together at the bottom of this fissure by the *corpus callosum,* a broad band of commissural fibers. The surface of each hemisphere is wrinkled by the presence of eminences known as *gyri* and furrows which are called *sulci,* or *fissures.* The fissures are deeper than sulci and can be recognized internally by corresponding indentations of the ventricles of the brain. A layer of cerebral cortex 1.3 to 4.5 mm thick covers the expansive surface of the cerebrum. It is estimated to contain 14 billion nerve cells.

There are two major grooves on the lateral surface of the brain. The *lateral fissure (of Sylvius)* begins as a deep cleft on the basal surface of the brain and extends laterally, posteriorly, and upward (Fig. 1). The *central sulcus (of Rolando)* runs from the dorsal border of the hemisphere near its midpoint obliquely downward and forward until it nearly meets the lateral fissure. For descriptive purposes the hemisphere is divided into four lobes. The *frontal lobe* (approximately the anterior one-third of the hemisphere) is the portion which is rostral to the central sulcus and above the lateral fissure. The *occipital lobe* is that part lying behind an arbitrary line drawn from the parieto-occipital fissure to the preoccipital notch. This lobe occupies a small area of the lateral surface but has more extensive territory on the medial aspect of the hemisphere. The *parietal lobe* extends from the central sulcus to the parieto-occipital fissure and is separated from the *temporal lobe* below by an imagi-

3

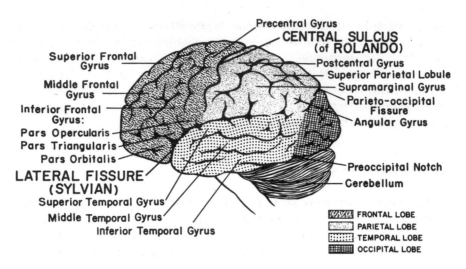

FIGURE 1. Lateral view of the brain.

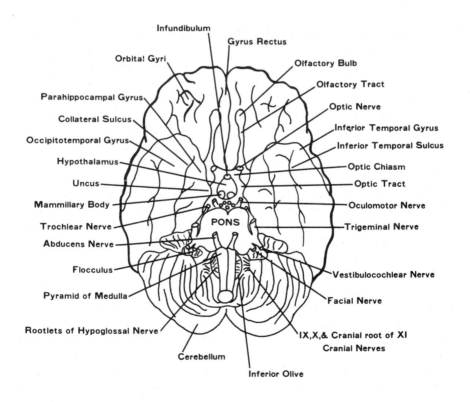

FIGURE 2. Ventral view of the brain.

4

nary line projected from the horizontal portion of the lateral fissure to the middle of the line demarking the occipital lobe. The gyri are subdivided areas roughly marked out by sulci whose patterns may show considerable individual variation. Figures 2 and 3 depict the structures that are located on the ventral and medial (midsagittal) surfaces of the brain.

The Brain Stem

The brain stem consists of the following areas of the brain: *medulla, pons, midbrain,* and *diencephalon*. This region is described in Chapter 9.

The Spinal Cord

With respect to the spinal cord, the terms *posterior* and *dorsal* are used interchangeably. Similarly, the terms *anterior* and *ventral* are interchangeable. Technically, the terms posterior and anterior should be employed in referring to the human spinal cord and dorsal and ventral to that of the quadruped.

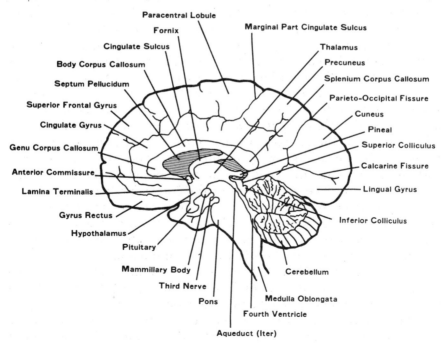

FIGURE 3. Medial (midsagittal) view of the brain.

The spinal cord is a slender cylinder surrounded by the closely applied *pia mater*. A *dural sac*, lined on the inner surface with the arachnoid membrane, encloses a liberal amount of cerebrospinal fluid which occupies the *subarachnoid space*. The spinal cord is anchored to the dura mater by paired lateral septa of the pia mater—the *denticulate ligaments*. The spinal cord is moderately enlarged in the cervical region and again in the lumbar region where nerve fibers supplying the upper and lower extremities are connected. Spinal nerves are attached to the spinal cord in pairs: 8 cervical; 12 thoracic; 5 lumbar; 5 sacral; and 1 coccygeal. Each spinal nerve has dorsal and ventral roots which form nearly continuous rows along the cord. The spinal cord does not extend to the lower end of the vertebral canal but ends at the level of the lower border of the first lumbar vertebra in a tapered cone, the *conus medullaris*. The pia mater continues caudally as a connective tissue filament, the *filum terminale*, which is attached to the periosteum of the coccyx. Since the cord is some 25 cm shorter than the vertebral column, the lumbar and sacral nerves require very long intervertebral roots extending from the cord to the intervertebral foramina where dorsal and ventral roots are joined. These roots descend in a bundle from the conus, and, from its resemblance to the tail of a horse, the formation is known as the *cauda equina*. Because of the difference in their lengths, the segments of the spinal cord are not aligned opposite corresponding segments of the vertebral column (Fig. 4).

In the transverse section the spinal cord is shown as an H, or butterfly-shaped area of gray substance with surrounding white substance made up of longitudinal nerve fibers (Fig. 5). Midline grooves are present on the dorsal and ventral surfaces—the *posterior median sulcus* and the *anterior median fissure*. The lateral surface contains a *posterolateral* and a *anterolateral sulcus*. These markings divide the white matter of the spinal cord into *posterior, lateral,* and *anterior funiculi*. The dorsal root zone is interposed between the posterior and lateral funiculi; the ventral root zone between the lateral and anterior funiculi. The gray matter of the cord contains posterior and anterior enlargements known respectively as the *posterior gray horns* and the *anterior gray horns*. Small *intermediolateral gray columns* are also present in the thoracic and upper lumbar segments of the spinal cord. The *nucleus dorsalis* (the dorsal nucleus of Clarke) has a similar distribution (C8 to L2) but is more prominent in its caudal extent. In the cervical and lumbosacral enlargements, the anterior horns are larger than in the thoracic segments. This is due to the fact that the muscle mass of the extremities is greater than that of the trunk and requires more anterior horn cells. Accordingly, the anterior horn of the lumbosacral enlargement is more massive than that of the

6

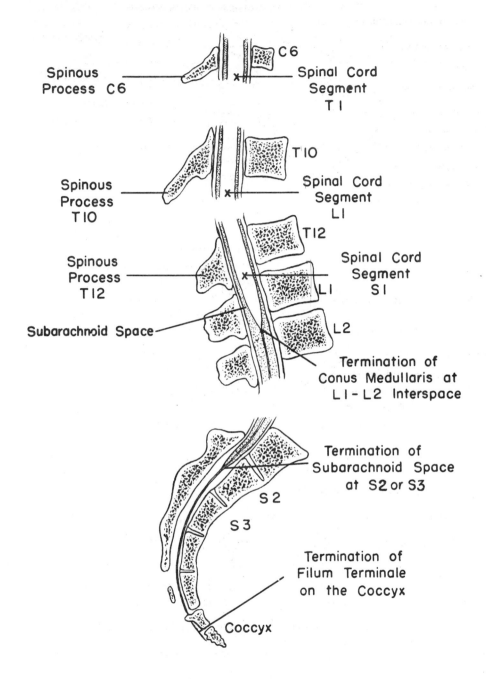

Spinous Process C6 —— × C6 —— Spinal Cord Segment T I

Spinous Process T10 —— × T10 Spinal Cord Segment L1

Spinous Process T12 —— × T12 L1 Spinal Cord Segment S1

Subarachnoid Space —— L2

Termination of Conus Medullaris at L1 – L2 Interspace

Termination of Subarachnoid Space at S2 or S3

S2

S3

Termination of Filum Terminale on the Coccyx

Coccyx

FIGURE 4. Diagram showing the relationship of certain structures of the spinal cord to the bodies and spinous processes of vertebrae.

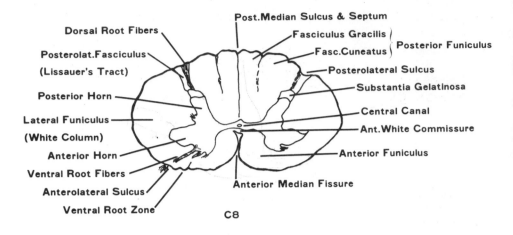

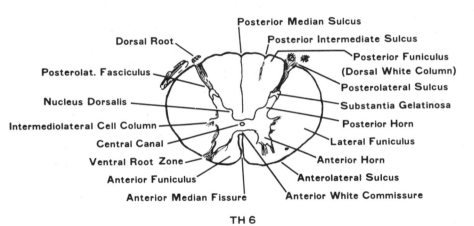

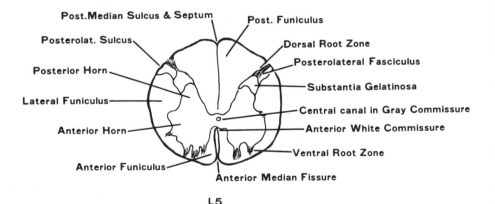

FIGURE 5. Cross sections of the spinal cord.

cervical enlargement because of the greater muscle mass in the lower extremity. With respect to the enlargements, note that there is a larger amount of white matter at the cervical level than at the lumbosacral region.

The gray matter of the cord can be subdivided into 9 *laminae of Rexed* (Fig. 6) on the basis of cytoarchitectonics and the longitudinal organization of the neurons. It is important to learn the general location of these laminae with respect to the overall configuration of the gray matter. Such information is essential in order to understand the functional significance of the origin and termination of the ascending and descending pathways. Laminae I through VI are confined to the posterior horn and are particularly concerned with the sensory input to the cord. Descending motor pathways also influence these laminae. Lamina II corresponds to the *substantia gelatinosa*. Lamina VII is located in the intermediate gray area and extends into the anterior horn. It contains both the *nucleus dorsalis* and the *intermediolateral gray column*. Lamina VIII is located in the anterior horn and contains many neurons that send axons (*commissural*) to the opposite side. Lamina IX is broken up into groups and is restricted to the anterior horn. It contains the *alpha* and *gamma* motor neurons that send axons into the ventral root of the spinal cord.

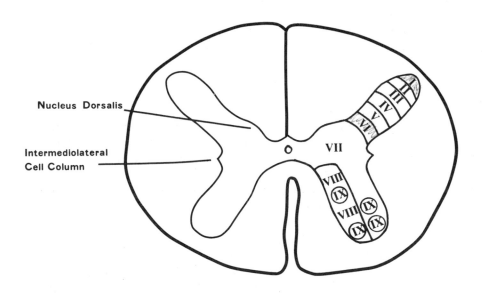

Nucleus Dorsalis

Intermediolateral
Cell Column

FIGURE 6. Rexed's laminae of the spinal cord gray matter.

9

2
Functional Components of the Spinal Nerves

The function of the nerves of the body may be conveniently categorized by the following method: the fibers which innervate the body wall are designated as *somatic*; those that innervate the viscera are termed *visceral*; *sensory* fibers are designated *afferent*, while *motor* fibers are classified as *efferent*.

Resumé of Functional Components

A. General afferent fibers

These are the sensory fibers which have their cells of origin located in the *dorsal root ganglia*.

1. *Somatic afferent* (GSA)

Includes the fibers which carry the exteroceptive (pain, temperature, and touch) and the proprioceptive impulses from sensory endings in the body wall, tendons, and joints.

2. *Visceral afferent* (GVA)

Are the fibers that carry sensory impulses from the visceral structures within the body.

B. General efferent fibers

1. *Somatic efferent* (GSE)

Consists of the motor fibers (originating from alpha and gamma motor-neurons of lamina IX) that innervate the striated musculature derived from the myotomes of somites.

2. *Visceral efferent* (GVE)

Consists of the autonomic fibers which innervate smooth

and cardiac muscle and regulate glandular secretion. *Preganglionic sympathetic* cell bodies are located in the intermediolateral cell column extending from C8 or T1 to L2 (lamina VII). *Preganglionic parasympathetic* cell bodies are located in a similar region in the sacral cord (S2 to S4).

CLASSIFICATION OF NERVE FIBERS

Nerve fibers can be categorized according to fiber diameter, degree of myelinization (thickness of the myelin sheath), and speed of conduction of the nerve impulse. In general, *the greater the diameter of the fiber, the thicker the myelin sheath, the faster the conduction velocity.* Currently, two classifications of nerve fibers are in use. One, which refers to groups I through IV, considers only sensory fibers, whereas the other, which refers to types A, B, and C, includes both sensory and motor fibers. Table 1 summarizes the two classifications.

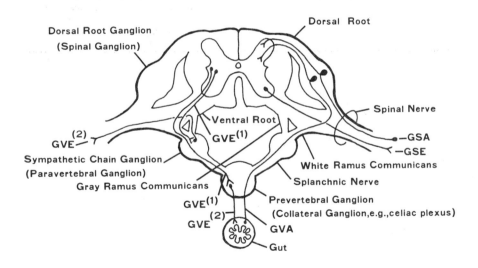

FIGURE 7. Components of spinal nerves, dorsal and ventral roots, and the sympathetic nervous system. Diagram of a typical thoracic spinal cord cross section. GVE [1] = preganglionic sympathic neuron, general visceral efferent; GVE [2] = postganglionic sympathetic neuron.

11

Table 1. Motor and Sensory Classification of Nerve Fibers

Sensory (Groups)	Sensory and Motor	Greatest Fiber Diameter (μ)	Greatest Conduction Velocity (meters/sec)	General Comments
Ia =	Aα	22	120	Motor—the large alpha motor neurons of lamina IX Sensory—the primary afferents (annulospiral) of muscle spindles
Ib =	Aα	22	120	Sensory—Golgi tendon organs, touch, and pressure receptors
II =	Aβ	13	70	Sensory—the secondary afferents (flower spray) of muscle spindles, touch, and pressure receptors, Pacinian corpuscles (vibratory sensors)
	Aγ	8	40	Motor—the small gamma motor neurons of lamina IX innervate muscle spindles
III =	Aδ	5	15	Sensory—small lightly myelinated fibers, touch, pressure, pain, and temperature
	B	3	14	Motor—small lightly myelinated preganglionic autonomic fibers
IV =	C	1	2	Motor—all postganglionic autonomic fibers (all are unmyelinated) Sensory—unmyelinated pain and temperature fibers

3
Spinal Reflexes and Muscle Tone

Spinal Reflexes

A reflex action consists of a specific, stereotyped motor response to an adequate sensory stimulus. The response may involve movement and/or glandular secretion. It may involve only two neurons (*simple, monosynaptic reflex arc*) as in the *myotatic knee-jerk*, or, as in most instances, it may utilize several to many additional neurons (*interneurons or internuncial cells*). A reflex may involve (1) just one or a few spinal cord levels (*segmental reflexes*), (2) several to many spinal cord levels (*intersegmental reflexes*), or (3) structures in the brain that influence the spinal cord (*supraspinal reflexes*).

Alpha and Gamma Motor Neurons

Muscle movement is the motor response to most reflexes that are tested clinically. In the final analysis this must involve the *facilitation* or *inhibition* of the alpha and gamma motor neurons of lamina IX.

Alpha motor neurons are the largest of the anterior horn cells. They can be stimulated monosynaptically by (1) the Ia primary afferents (annulospiral endings) of the muscle spindles, (2) a small percentage of the corticospinal tract fibers, and (3) possibly by a small percentage of the lateral vestibulospinal tract fibers. Most of the stimulation of these neurons occurs through interneurons in response to segmental, intersegmental, and supraspinal reflexes. All

13

of the descending tracts of the spinal cord ultimately influence the activity of these neurons. The alpha motor neurons innervate GSA, the large *extrafusal skeletal muscle fibers*. Through *recurrent collaterals*, they also excite one type of interneuron called the *Renshaw cell*, which then inhibits the alpha motor neurons (*negative feedback*).

Gamma motor neurons differ from the alpha motor neurons in that they are (1) smaller, (2) not excited monosynaptically, and (3) not involved in inhibitory feedback mechanisms by the Renshaw cells. Most of the descending pathways of the spinal cord influence their activity. Considerable control is exerted on the gamma neurons directly by the reticular system and indirectly by the cerebellum and basal ganglia.

Muscle Spindles

Muscle spindles are encapsulated structures 3 to 4 mm in length located, in varying numbers, in most skeletal muscles of the body. They are particularly numerous in the small delicate muscles of the hand. The spindles consist of several fibers of modified striated muscle (Fig. 8). Because they are enclosed in the fusiform shaped

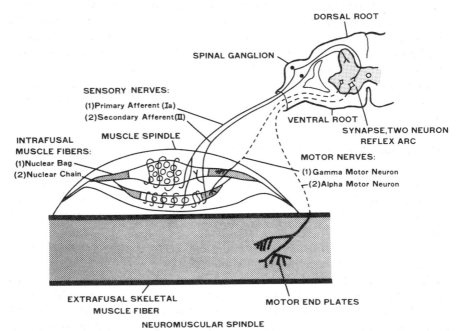

Figure 8

14

spindle, they are referred to as *intrafusal muscle fibers* in contrast to the large extrafusal fibers. The spindle is attached at both ends to an extrafusal fiber. Consequently, the entire structure is *parallel* to the extrafusal fiber which becomes quite significant when considering the function of this structure. There are two types of intrafusal fibers. Both have striations near their ends but lack them in the center where there is an abundance of sarcoplasm and cell nuclei. In one type, the cell nuclei are clustered into a "bag-like" structure and thus are called the *nuclear bag* intrafusal fiber. The other contains a single row of nuclei and is called the *nuclear chain* fiber. Both types of fibers are *innervated by the gamma motor neurons* and supplied with sensory nerve endings. The very large group Ia fibers (see Table 1) innervate both types of fibers and are referred to as *primary afferents* (or in the older terminology, the annulospiral endings). The nuclear chain fibers and, to a lesser extent, the nuclear bag fibers are also supplied by group II afferents (*secondary endings*, or in the older terminology, the flower spray endings).

Muscle Tonus

A normal, live muscle which appears to be fully relaxed still possesses a small amount of tension. If it is palpated in a resting state, the muscle will be found to have a quality of resilience rather than complete flabbiness. When it is passively stretched by moving one of the joints, a certain amount of resistance will be encountered in the muscle which is not related to any conscious effort on the part of the patient. These characteristics — subdued activity at rest, and involuntary reaction opposing mechanical stretch — are the chief clinical manifestations of muscle tonus.

A muscle loses its tonus at once if the ventral roots containing its motor nerve fibers are cut. Tonus is likewise abolished by cutting the dorsal nerve roots that contain sensory fibers from the muscle. These familiar experiments indicate that tonus of the sort that has been described is maintained and regulated in muscles by reflex activity of the nervous system, and is not a property of isolated muscle.

The Stretch Reflex

The stretch reflex is the basic neural mechanism for maintaining tonus in muscles. Aside from its role in keeping relaxed muscles slightly active, the stretch reflex is capable of increasing the tension of selected muscle groups to provide a background of postural muscle tonus on which voluntary movements are superimposed.

The stretch (myotatic) reflex can be tested by tapping the patellar tendon. This stretches the quadriceps femoris muscle. Since the muscle spindles are in parallel with the extrafusal fibers of the quadriceps, they will also be stretched. This stretching will stimulate the sensory endings in the spindle, in particular the primary afferents (Ia). The latter neurons monosynaptically stimulate the alpha motor neurons that supply the quadriceps and polysynaptically inhibit the antagonistic muscles. Consequently, the quadriceps will suddenly contract causing the leg to extend.

The *function of the intrafusal fibers is to inform the nervous system of the length and rate of change in length of the extrafusal fibers.* The primary afferents are related to both length and rate of change in length, whereas the secondary endings (II) are primarily length detectors. Much of the information from the spindles is utilized at supraspinal centers (for example, cerebellum and cerebral cortex). These centers can directly and indirectly influence the descending pathways that facilitate and inhibit the alpha and gamma motor neurons. Finally, the *gamma motor neurons can bias the sensitivity of the muscle spindle by causing the intrafusal fibers to contract.* When an external load is applied to a muscle, this *gamma-loop* system tends to keep the muscle at constant length.

Golgi Tendon Organs

These are encapsulated structures located in series with the large collagenous fibers of tendons near the muscle insertion and, thus, are *in series with the extrafusal muscle fibers.* Within the capsule, sensory nerve endings (*Ib afferents*) terminate in small bundles of collagenous fibers of tendons. The Golgi tendon organs are primarily *tension recorders* and respond to active contraction of the muscle. They *polysynaptically inhibit the agonists and facilitate the antagonistic muscles.* This is responsible for the *clasp-knife phenomenon* in *upper motor neuronal lesions* in which there is a sudden release of a spastic muscle under forced stretch.

The Flexor and Crossed Extension Reflexes

These are examples of *protective reflexes.* If a cat places one foot on something very hot, the animal will reflexly withdraw that extremity. This is an example of the *flexor reflex* (withdrawal reflex) and involves noxious stimuli which polysynaptically facilitate the alpha motor neurons to the ipsilateral flexor muscles and inhibit those to the extensors. Simultaneously, a *crossed extension reflex* will occur. The contralateral limb will be extended in order to support the weight of the body. Thus, contralateral flexors are inhibited while extensors are facilitated.

The Propriospinal System

Immediately surrounding the entire gray matter of the spinal cord is a narrow rim of white matter which is called the *fasciculus proprius* or the *propriospinal system*. This system mediates the long intersegmental spinal reflexes. The neurons traversing this system have their cell bodies located in one level of the spinal cord and send their axons to another. This pathway facilitates the coordination of upper and lower extremity movements both contralaterally and ipsilaterally.

4

The Descending Motor Pathways

THE MOTOR AREAS OF THE CEREBRAL CORTEX

The primary motor area, also known as Brodmann's area 4, is located in the precentral (or anterior central) gyrus of the frontal lobe (see Figs. 1 and 44). It forms a band extending from the lateral fissure upward to the dorsal border of the hemisphere and a short distance beyond on the medial surface of the frontal lobe in the rostral aspect of the paracentral lobule. The left motor strip controls the right side of the body. The larynx and tongue are represented in the lowest part of this strip, followed in upward sequence by the face, thumb, hand, forearm, arm, thorax, abdomen, thigh, calf, foot, and the muscles of the perineum. In humans, areas for the hand, tongue, and larynx are disproportionately large, conforming with the development of elaborate motor control. The spatial organization of the motor cortex resembles a map showing a distorted image of the body turned upside down and reversed left for right (Fig. 9). Immediately rostral to area 4 is the *premotor cortex* which consists of *areas 6 and 8*. Area 8 influences eye movements. The most medial aspect of area 6 can be observed on a midsagittal brain preparation just rostral to the paracentral lobule (see Fig. 3). This is the location of the *supplementary motor area*. A third motor area referred to as the *secondary motor area* is present on the most ventral aspect of the pre- and postcentral gyri. This overlaps the *secondary somatosensory cortex*.

18

THE PYRAMIDAL SYSTEM

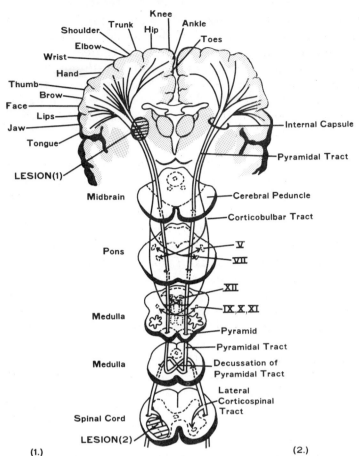

(1.)	(2.)
UPPER MOTOR NEURON	**LOWER MOTOR NEURON**
LESION	**LESION**
Contralateral Hemiparesis	Paresis Limited to Specific Muscle Groups
Postural Flexion of Arm, Extension of Leg	Gait Depends on Muscles Affected. Flail-like Movements Common
Muscles Hypertonic	Muscles Flaccid
Tendon Reflexes Hyperactive	Tendon Reflexes Absent or Hypoactive
Atrophy Not Prominent	Atrophy Prominent
No Muscle Fasciculations	Muscle Fasciculations Present
Pathological Reflexes Present	Contractures & Skeletal Deformities May Develop

FIGURE 9.

19

Descending Fibers From Motor Areas of the Cerebral Cortex

Skeletal muscle activity is the result of the net influence upon the alpha and gamma motor neurons of the spinal cord and upon the motor components of the cranial nerve nuclei. Collectively, *these are the neurons which provide the final direct link with muscles through myoneural junctions (motor end plates). Such neurons are referred to as lower motor neurons (LMN). Their cell bodies reside within the central nervous system and their axons make synaptic contact with extrafusal and intrafusal muscle fibers of somatic and branchiomeric origin.*

Lower motor neuronal activity is regulated by a number of descending motor pathways which either directly or indirectly are controlled by the cerebral cortex, cerebellum, or basal ganglia. In the strictest sense, the neurons in all such pathways should be referred to as *upper motor neurons (UMN). Upper motor neurons operate directly or through interneurons upon alpha and gamma motor neurons and upon motor components of the cranial nerve nuclei. They are contained completely within the central nervous system.* Clinicians usually use the term UMN only when referring to the corticospinal tract, or to a lesser extent the corticobulbar tract (see Fig. 9).

Motor pathways that arise from the cerebral cortex include the following:

1. *Corticospinal System* (see Fig. 9)

   This is also referred to as the *pyramidal tract system.* It was formerly considered to be the pathway that initiated and controlled all "voluntary" muscular activity. It is now known that it is *primarily concerned with skilled movements of the distal extremities and in particular with facilitation of the alpha and gamma motor neurons that innervate distal flexor musculature.* Approximately a third of the fibers in this system arise from area 4, the primary motor cortex, and about 3 per cent of these fibers originate from the large pyramidal cells (Betz cells) located in the fifth layer of the cortex. Another third of the fibers arise from area 6, and the remainder of the fibers originate from the parietal lobe (primarily areas 1, 2, and 3). The pathway passes through the posterior limb of the internal capsule, middle of the cerebral cerebri, breaks up into bundles in the basilar portion of the pons, and then collects into a discrete bundle in the pyramids of the medulla. *This system was originally named the pyramidal tract because of its passage through the medullary pyramid,* and not because of its origin from pyramidal cells in the cortex. In the lower levels of the medulla, the corticospinal tract crosses (decussates) to the opposite

20

side (a region referred to as the *level of the motor or pyramidal tract decussation*). Approximately 90 per cent of the fibers cross at this level and become the *lateral corticospinal tract* which passes to all cord levels in the lateral funiculus and synapses in the lateral aspect of laminae IV through VIII. A small percentage of the fibers (perhaps those arising from Betz cells) synapse directly upon the alpha and gamma motor neurons in lamina IX. A small percentage of the fibers do not decussate and descend in the anterior funiculus of the cervical and upper thoracic cord levels as the *anterior corticospinal tract.* However, this pathway decussates through the anterior white commissure prior to entering and synapsing upon cells in lamina VIII. The number of fibers in both tracts decreases in successively lower cord segments as more and more fibers reach their terminations. *It is of interest that the corticospinal tract is not purely motor.* It also sends fibers to synapse in the nuclei gracilis and cuneatus, which are sensory relay nuclei, and additionally terminates on interneurons in laminae IV, V, and VI. These interneurons mediate local reflex arcs as well as give rise to ascending sensory pathways. Thus, it appears as though *the cerebral cortex apparently can modify its own sensory input.*

2. *Corticobulbar Tract* (see Fig. 9)

The fibers of the corticobulbar tract start out in company with the corticospinal tract but take a divergent route at the level of the midbrain. A few of the fibers continue along with the corticospinal system in the pyramids. This pathway terminates in the brain stem on motor nuclei of cranial nerve V (trigeminal); VII (facial); IX, X, and XI (glossopharyngeal, vagus, and accessory); and XII (hypoglossal). In each instance, only those motor nuclei that innervate striated skeletal musculature either of somatic or branchiomeric origin are concerned. With the exception of that portion of the facial nucleus that innervates facial musculature below the angle of the eye, all of the nuclei are bilaterally innervated. The lower facial nucleus receives a crossed component only. Clinical evidence indicates that sometimes the hypoglossal nucleus receives a crossed component only.

3. *Corticotectal Tract*

In the past, some authors have referred to the pathways that arise from the cerebral cortex (from areas 6, 8, 17, 18, and 19) to influence extraocular muscle movement as corticomesencephalic tracts. Some even included them as part of the corticobulbar system. Many of the fibers synapse in the tectum of the superior colliculus, the interstitial nucleus of Cajal, or the nucleus of

21

Darkschewitch. These nuclei may project their fibers into the medial longitudinal fasciculus (MLF) to synapse upon the oculomotor, trochlear, and abducens nuclei. The picture may even be more complex in that the cortical fibers may first synapse in various regions of the reticular system (gaze centers in the pontine region have been suggested). The reticular system may project into the medial longitudinal fasciculus to innervate the extrinsic eye muscle nuclei.

4. *Corticorubrospinal System*

   This represents an indirect route from the cerebral cortex to the spinal cord. Many of the fibers that originate with the corticospinal system as the *corticorubral tract* project to the ipsilateral red nucleus in the tegmentum of the midbrain. The red nucleus gives rise to the *rubrospinal tract,* a crossed pathway, that passes just anterior to the lateral corticospinal tract in the lateral funiculus to all cord levels. It synapses in the lateral aspect of laminae V, VI, and VII and thus overlaps part of the termination of the corticospinal tract. In fact, it is functionally similar to the latter tract in that it facilitates flexor alpha and gamma motor neurons and inhibits extensors. It is important to realize that the red nucleus is also a way–station between the cerebellum and the ventral lateral nucleus of the thalamus.

5. *Corticoreticulospinal System*

   The reticular formation of the brain stem receives a large input from *corticoreticular tracts* that accompany the corticospinal tract. Two areas of the reticular formation send major projections into the spinal cord. The medial aspect of the pontine reticular formation gives rise to the uncrossed *pontine (medial) reticulospinal tract.* This pathway travels in the brain stem just anterior to the medial longitudinal fasciculus and passes through the anterior funiculus to all cord levels to synapse in laminae VIII and VII. This tract is mainly *facilitatory for extensor motor neurons. The reticular system is the most important drive of the gamma system.* The medial aspect of the medullary reticular formation also gives rise to the *medullary (lateral) reticulospinal tract* that is primarily uncrossed (with a small crossed component). This tract passes to all cord levels in the lateral funiculus just anterior to the rubrospinal tract. There is controversy regarding the exact function of this pathway with respect to the alpha and gamma motor neurons. It synapses in laminae VII and IX. The tract conveys *autonomic information* from higher centers to the *intermediolateral cell column* to influence respiration, circulation, sweating, shivering, and dilation of the pupils.

Other Descending Motor Pathways

1. *Vestibulospinal Tracts*

   The vestibulospinal tracts are discussed in Chapter 14. Both of these pathways pass into the anterior funiculus and synapse upon cells in laminae VIII and VII. The *lateral vestibulospinal tract* extends the entire length of the cord and the *medial vestibulospinal tract* terminates at upper thoracic levels. *The lateral tract facilitates extensor alpha motor neurons and inhibits flexors.* Very little is known about the medial vestibulospinal tract in man.

2. *The Medial Longitudinal Fasciculus* (MLF)

   The MLF contains several pathways that project into the anterior funiculus of the spinal cord. It contains the *pontine reticulospinal tract* and the *medial vestibulospinal tract* which have already been discussed. In addition, it contains the *tectospinal tract* which arises from the superior colliculus, crosses to the opposite side near the oculomotor nucleus (in the dorsal tegmental decussation) to join the MLF. The *interstitiospinal tract* that arises from the interstitial nucleus of Cajal (an accessory oculomotor nucleus) is also part of the MLF. It supplies only the upper cervical levels where it synapses in laminae VIII and VII. This tract is concerned in neck and head reflex movement in response to visual stimuli.

GENERALIZATIONS CONCERNING THE INFLUENCE OF DESCENDING PATHWAYS UPON THE SPINAL CORD

Review Figure 6 with respect to the location of the laminae and their relation to the various descending pathways. With respect to the anterior horn, those pathways that pass through the anterior funiculus to the medial aspect of the gray matter (namely laminae VIII and VII) in general, tend to facilitate extensor activity and inhibit flexor activity (lateral vestibulospinal tract and the pontine reticulospinal tract). The pathways that synapse in the lateral aspect of the gray matter (namely laminae V, VI, and VII) tend to facilitate flexor activity and inhibit extensor activity (lateral corticospinal tract and the rubrospinal tract). Clinicians usually refer to the descending motor pathways other than the corticospinal system as the *extrapyramidal system* (indicating that they do not pass through the pyramids of the medulla).

5

The Anterolateral
System

The *anterolateral (ventrolateral) system* consists of a diffuse bundle of fibers located at the juncture of the anterior and lateral funiculi of the spinal cord. It contains pathways which, according to older terminology, are called the *lateral and anterior spinothalamic tracts*. This system conveys *pain, temperature, and tactile sensations*. The tactile components will be considered in Chapter 7.

THE PAIN-TEMPERATURE PATHWAYS

The clinical management of pain is a problem that continuously confronts the physician, yet there are wide gaps in our knowledge concerning the structure and physiology of the receptors and central pathways mediating this modality. The peripheral receptors for pain are presumably naked terminals of branching networks of fine nerve fibers. They are probably specialized chemoreceptors in that they are excited by tissue chemicals released in response to *noxious stimuli*. Pain fibers enter the spinal cord through the dorsal root zone and divide at once into short ascending and descending branches which run logitudinally in the *posterolateral fasciculus (Lissauer's tract)*. Within a segment or two they leave this tract to synapse with neurons in the posterior horn. The exact connections are not known; however, they probably synapse upon *interneurons* in laminae III and IV (not in lamina II, the substantia gelatinosa, as previously taught) which project primarily to laminae VI and VII to synapse upon the cells of origin of the *lateral spinothalamic tract*.

Information from multiple sensory and motor systems is processed

24

in laminae VI and VII. Many of the neurons in these laminae have axons which cross anterior to the central canal in the *anterior white commissure* and then course rostrally in the anterolateral system as the lateral spinothalamic component. This system extends through the spinal cord and brain stem supplying inputs to many regions of the *reticular formation* and several *thalamic nuclei* including *intralaminar nuclei*, the *posterior nuclear complex (PO)*, and the *ventral posterolateral nucleus VPL* (referred to by physiologists as part of the *ventrobasal complex*). *Thalamocortical fibers* relay pain in-

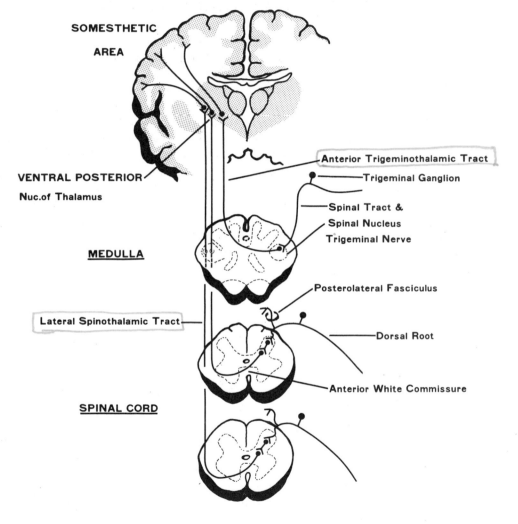

PAIN-TEMPERATURE

FIGURE 10

formation from the thalamic nuclei to primarily the *secondary somatic sensory area* of the cerebrum (Fig. 10). Possibly a few fibers conveying pain sensations from the VPL nucleus project to the primary somatic sensory area (3, 1, 2) of the postcentral gyrus (see Fig. 44).

The anterolateral system is phylogenetically old. It is predominantly a relatively slow-conducting, polysynaptic system. In man, a small percentage of the fibers go directly to the thalamus, but most synapse in the medial aspect of the reticular formation throughout its length in the brain stem to be integrated with autonomic nervous system components and other structures. Ascending reticular fibers, in turn, relay pain information to the thalamic nuclei outlined above and to the hypothalamus. The projection to the VPL nucleus is somatotopically organized so that the input from the upper body is located medial to that from the lower body.

Pain fibers from the face, the cornea of the eye, the sinuses and the mucosa of the lips, cheeks, and tongue are carried in the trigeminal nerve and its sensory ganglion (the semilunar, trigeminal, or gasserian ganglion). Upon entering the brain stem in the pontine region, these fibers form a descending tract—the *spinal tract of V*. Terminals of the spinal tract of the trigeminal nerve make synapses in an adjacent nucleus, the *nucleus of the spinal tract of V*. Axons originating in the nucleus of the spinal tract of V cross to the opposite side and ascend as the *anterior (ventral) trigeminothalamic tract* to the *ventral posteromedial nucleus (VPM)* of the thalamus. This pathway also sends fibers to synapse in the reticular formation and probably to the other thalamic nuclei (aside from VPL) that receive projections from the anterolateral system.

Perception of Pain

Two types of pain sensation are usually recognized. One is *fast pain (sharp, pricking)* with little emotional counterpart, and the other is *slow (burning)* and does have emotional components that evoke aversive behavior. The former is conveyed by lightly myelinated A-delta and unmyelinated C fibers (see Table 1). Evidence indicates that the central nervous system processes the two types of pain sensation separately. *Apparently fast pain is projected directly to the thalamus through the lateral spinothalamic component of the anterolateral system and is somatotopically arranged,* accounting for the ability to sharply localize such pain. On the other hand, *slow pain fibers in the anterolateral system synapse in the brain stem reticular formation which relays the information to the thalamic and hypo-*

26

thalamic structures integrated with emotional behavior. The pathways associated with slow pain are not organized to provide discrete spatial or temporal information.

The descending pathways from the cerebral cortex and other supraspinal structures can synapse upon nerve cell bodies related to the relay of pain in the posterior horn or reticular formation and modify the pain sensations. Other somatic sensory pathways can also influence the neurons involved in the transfer of pain information. This provides so-called *gate-controlled mechanisms by which emotional behavior and various sensory modalities can influence pain.* A soldier in the heat of battle may not experience pain as a result of severe injury whereas under different conditions the same injury may evoke unbearable pain. *Acupuncture anesthesia* and surgery performed under *hypnosis* can perhaps be explained on the basis of this "gate" theory.

Painful stimuli are recognized consciously when nerve impulses arrive at the thalamus. In man, the posterior and intralaminar nuclei must be destroyed in order to relieve intractable pain. Destruction of the cerebral cortical projection areas does not eliminate pain. Other qualities besides the crude perception of pain as such are not appreciated by the thalamus but are supplied by the parietal cortex, where pain stimuli are integrated with other sensory stimuli.

Temperature Sense

The receptors in the skin for the sense of cold and warmth probably consist of both naked and encapsulated endings. The fibers and cells serving the sensory path for temperature perception follow the same course as those of the pain pathway. The two systems are so closely associated in the central nervous system that they can scarcely be distinguished anatomically, and an injury to one usually affects the other to a similar degree. Testing either pain or temperature sensibility accomplishes the same result. If pain sense is normal, pricking the skin with a sharp point is reported as feeling "sharp" rather than "dull," or tubes filled with warm and cool water may be applied to the skin to determine whether differences in temperature can be felt.

Effect of Cutting the Lateral Spinothalamic Tract

The lateral spinothalamic tracts are sometimes sectioned in humans to relieve intractable pain—a surgical procedure known as

27

tractotomy. The cut is made in the anterior part of the lateral funiculus. Some damage is done to the anterior spinocerebellar tract, and perhaps to certain extrapyramidal motor fibers, but no permanent symptoms are produced except a loss of pain sensibility on the contralateral side, beginning one or two segments below the cut. In some patients pain is only temporarily relieved suggesting that other routes may be available or that the information is mediated by both crossed and uncrossed tracts. Bilateral tractotomy is usually necessary to abolish pain from visceral organs.

Sensory Effects of Dorsal Root Irritation

Mechanical compression, or local inflammation, of dorsal nerve roots irritates pain fibers and commonly produces pain which is felt along the anatomical distribution of the roots affected. The area of skin supplied by one dorsal root is a dermatome, or skin segment. The approximate boundaries of human dermatomes are shown in Figure 11. Pain which is limited in distribution to one or more dermatomes is known as radicular pain.

Sensory changes other than pain may be associated with dorsal root irritation. There may be localized areas of parasthesia, such as spontaneous sensations of prickling, tingling, or numbness. Zones of hyperesthesia, in which tactile stimuli appear to be grossly exaggerated, may be present. If the pathological process is a progressive one which gradually destroys fibers, the dorsal roots will finally lose their ability to conduct sensory impulses. There will be hypesthesia (diminished sensitivity) and eventually anesthesia (the complete absence of all forms of sensibility).

Visceral Pain — Referred Pain

The parenchyma of internal organs, including the brain itself, is not supplied with pain receptors. The walls of arteries, all peritoneal surfaces, pleural membranes, and the dura mater covering the brain may be sources of severe pain, especially when they are subjected to inflammation or mechanical traction. Abnormal contraction or dilation of the walls of hollow viscera also causes pain.

Pain of visceral origin is apt to be vaguely localized. At times it is felt in a surface area of the body far removed from its actual source, a phenomenon known as referred pain. For example: the pain of coronary heart disease may be felt in the chest wall, left axilla, or down the inside of the left arm; inflammation of the peritoneum

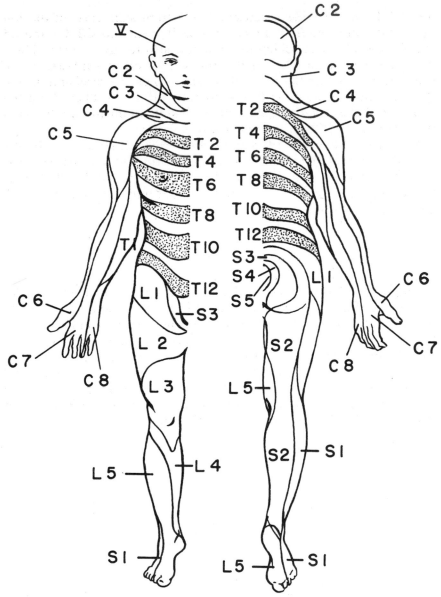

FIGURE 11. Segmental areas of innervation of the skin. Overlapping of one segment occurs between adjacent dermatomes.

covering the diaphragm may be felt over the shoulder. In each case, the neurons that supply the skin area in which the pain is felt enter the same segment of the spinal cord as do the neurons which actually conduct the pain stimuli from the visceral organ. Spinal cord seg-

29

ments T1 and T2 receive sensory fibers from skin areas of the left upper extremity and from the heart as well; segments C3, C4 and C5 supply the skin of the shoulder area and also receive sensory fibers from the diaphragm. One of the many theoretical explanations of referred pain is that the visceral sensory fibers are discharging into the same pool of neurons in the spinal cord as the fibers from the skin, and that an overflow of impulses results in misinterpretation of the true origin of the pain by the sensory cortex.

Pain may also be referred from deep somatic structures. In the case of ligaments and muscles associated with the vertebral column, the referred area is not always in the same segmental distribution as the level of origin of the pain impulses. Pain impulses from the teeth may also be referred.

Pain Reflexes

The sudden jerking away of the hand after accidental contact with a very hot object is a familiar example of a pain reflex. To operate this reflex, axons of cells of the posterior horn serve as intermediary links between sensory and motor neurons, passing up and down the spinal cord for several segments in order to make the appropriate lower motor neuron connections. These internuncial neurons and other intraspinal neurons connecting different segments of the cord contribute fibers to the fasciculus proprius, a zone of white matter that lies next to the gray substance of the spinal cord.

6

Proprioception and Stereognosis

THE DORSAL ROOTS AND DORSAL ROOT ZONES OF THE SPINAL CORD

The dorsal roots of the spinal cord consist almost entirely of sensory or afferent nerve fibers. All stimuli from the skin, and from internal structures as well, must pass through them to reach the spinal cord. The cell bodies of these fibers are located in spinal ganglia. Each ganglion cell possesses a single nerve process which divides like a "T," with a central branch running to the spinal cord and a peripheral branch coming from a receptor organ. There are no synapses in a spinal ganglion.

The area in which the dorsal root fibers enter the spinal cord, in the region of the dorsolateral sulcus, is called the dorsal root zone. Although there is a tendency for the largest and most heavily myelinated fibers to occupy the most medial position in this zone, there is considerable intermingling of large and small fibers.

Many of the large calibered fibers are proprioceptive fibers coming chiefly from neuromuscular and neurotendinous spindles; some come from Pacinian corpuscles and other encapsulated receptors between muscles and in joint capsules. The proprioceptive fibers conduct sensory impulses from muscles, tendons, ligaments, and joints. These messages are essential for awareness of the position of the limbs and their movements, often referred to as the kinesthetic sense. Most proprioceptive impulses which reach the central nervous system are not directed to the sensory perception centers of the brain; instead they are distributed to other areas which do not func-

31

tion at a conscious level. The unconscious subdivision of the proprioceptive system is concerned with mechanisms of automatic motor control and is primarily related to the cerebellum.

Pathways of Proprioception in the Spinal Cord and Brain

After entering the spinal cord, proprioceptive fibers continue without synaptic interruption in at least three divergent routes (Fig. 12).

1. *Direct Fibers to Lower Motor Neurons in the Anterior Gray Horns*

   These are the afferent fibers of the two neurons that make up the stretch reflex arc. They arise within a muscle spindle and end by synapse with motor cells within one or two spinal segments of the level at which they enter the spinal cord.

2. *Fibers to Spinocerebellar Pathways*

   Some proprioceptive fiber collaterals (primarily from Ia and Ib afferents) as well as fibers conveying other sensory modalities such as touch and pressure, synapse with neurons in the base of the posterior horn of the cord. The posterior funicular gray nucleus (laminae V, VI, and VII) in the lumbar and sacral levels, send crossed and uncrossed fibers to the *anterior spinocerebellar* tract which is the most peripheral tract in the ventral margin of the lateral funiculus. The *nucleus dorsalis* or *Clarke's nucleus* (lamina VII), located in the base of the posterior horn (T1 and L2), sends ipsilateral fibers rostrally in the *posterior spinocerebellar tract* which is located just posterior to the *anterior spinocerebellar tract* in the lateral funiculus. The posterior and anterior spinocerebellar pathways are primarily concerned with the lower extremities. The former pathway provides information concerning individual extremity muscles, whereas the latter relays information concerning the status of the entire extremity. Some collateral fibers from the levels of C1 to T5 synapse with neurons in the *accessory cuneate nucleus* to form ipsilateral *cuneocerebellar tract* or *dorsal arcuate fibers*, which is the upper extremity counterpart to the posterior spinocerebellar tract. All of the above tracts terminate primarily in the vermis of the cerebellum. The posterior spinocerebellar and cuneocerebellar tracts enter the cerebellum through the inferior cerebellar peduncle. The anterior spinocerebellar tract takes a separate course and enters the cerebellum through the superior cerebellar peduncle. These tracts report the instantaneous activity of muscle groups to the cerebellum. The latter is thus capable of modifying the action of the muscle

32

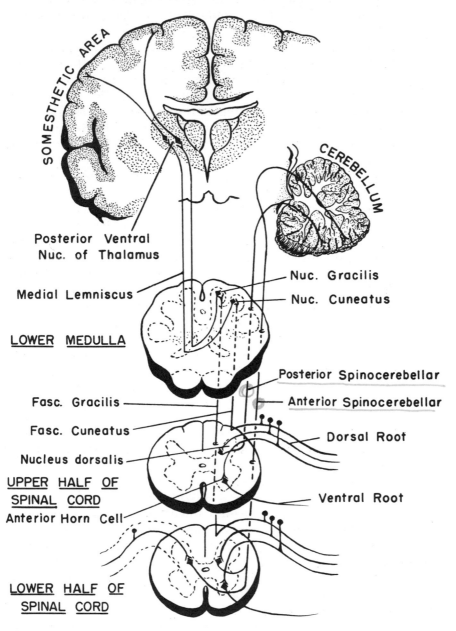

SOMESTHETIC AREA

CEREBELLUM

Posterior Ventral
Nuc. of Thalamus

Nuc. Gracilis

Nuc. Cuneatus

Medial Lemniscus

LOWER MEDULLA

Posterior Spinocerebellar

Anterior Spinocerebellar

Fasc. Gracilis

Fasc. Cuneatus

Dorsal Root

Nucleus dorsalis

UPPER HALF OF
SPINAL CORD

Ventral Root

Anterior Horn Cell

LOWER HALF OF
SPINAL CORD

PROPRIOCEPTION-STEREOGNOSIS

FIGURE 12.

33

groups so that the movements are smoothly and accurately *performed. The forelimb equivalent of the anterior spino-cerebellar tract is the rostral spinocerebellar tract.*

3. *Fibers Turning Directly Upward in the Posterior Funiculus* The fibers which form the first link of a pathway to the cerebrum arise from receptors in the connective tissue near joints for position sense. Recent evidence suggests that proprioceptive fibers from neuromuscular (Ia fibers) and Golgi tendon organs (Ib fibers) may also project through this system to the thalamus. Formerly, it was thought that all such proprioceptive information traveled primarily to the cerebellum. These fibers ascend in the posterior funiculi of the spinal cord to relay nuclei in the lower part of the medulla. Fibers from the leg ascend adjacent to the dorsal median septum and form the *fasciculus gracilis.* Fibers from the arm ascend lateral to the leg fibers and constitute the *fasciculus cuneatus.* Both fasciculi ascend to the lower medulla where they terminate in the *nucleus gracilis* and *nucleus cuneatus*, respectively. Clinicians often refer to these tracts as the posterior or *dorsal column pathways* and to the nuclei as the *dorsal column nuclei* (DCN). Fibers from the cells of these nuclei promptly cross to the opposite side in the decussation of the medial lemniscus. They then ascend as the *medial lemniscus* to the thalamus and terminate in the *ventral posterolateral* (VPL) *nucleus. In contrast to the anterolateral system discussed in the last chapter, few, if any, of the fibers in this system synapse in the reticular formation.* It is a phylogenetically more recent system. Thalamocortical fibers from this relay center continue to the *postcentral gyrus* of the parietal lobe. The band of the cortex which receives these terminals has been designated as the somesthetic area. The topographic representation of the body areas in this region is similar to that of the motor strip which lies parallel with it on the opposite side of the central sulcus. The conscious recognition of body and limb posture requires cortical participation.

In addition to fibers of proprioception, other fibers concerned with certain aspects of the senses of touch and pressure travel in the posterior funiculi, medial lemnisci, and thalamus to the postcentral gyri. This pathway to the cerebral cortex is necessary for *tactile discrimination:* the ability to appreciate two separate points at which pressure is applied simultaneously; to recognize the size, shape, and texture of objects by feeling; and to identify letters and figures drawn on the skin by touch. Such faculty is known as *stereognosis*, the ability to recognize form; its absence is designated as *astereognosis.* Vibratory sensation is also conveyed through this pathway.

Disturbances of Sensation Following Interruption of the Proprioceptive Pathways

Lesions which damage the conscious proprioceptive pathway produce defects in muscle sense and in stereognosis. The symptoms seem to be more prominent after injury of the posterior funiculi, but they are also found, in varying degrees, with lesions of the gracile and cuneate nuclei, the medial lemniscus, thalamus, or postcentral gyrus. A patient with bilateral posterior funiculus damage suffers ataxia (loss of muscular coordination) which causes a marked disturbance of gait. Unless he can watch the movements of the limbs and voluntarily correct errors, he stumbles, staggers, and may fall.

Clinical signs of injury to the funiculus frequently tested in a neurological examination are:

1. Inability to Recognize Limb Position.

   The patient is unable to say, without looking, whether a joint is put in a position of flexion or extension.

2. Astereognosis.

   There is loss, or impairment, of the ability to recognize common objects, such as keys, coins, blocks, and marbles by touching and handling them with the eyes closed.

3. Loss of Two Point Discrimination.

   There is loss of the normal facility of recognizing two points simultaneously applied to the skin as distinct from one single point. The two points of a compass may be used for testing.

4. Loss of Vibratory Sense.

   A vibrating tuning fork applied by the base to a bony prominence is normally perceived as a "buzzy," mildly tingling sensation. When this ability is lost, the patient cannot differentiate between a vibrating fork and a silent one.

5. Positive Romberg Sign.

   In this test the patient is asked to stand with the feet placed close together. The amount of body sway is noted while the eyes are open, then compared with the degree of sway present with the eyes closed. An abnormal accentuation of sway or an actual loss of balance with the eyes closed is a positive result. Visual sense is able to compensate, in part, for a deficiency in conscious recognition of muscle and joint position. Therefore, the patient may be able to maintain his balance if he is allowed to open his eyes. Symptoms of ataxia caused by lesions of the cerebellum are, on the contrary, not corrected by visual compensation.

7

Tactile Senses

Under ordinary circumstances tactile sensations are complex in nature since they involve the blending of a number of more elementary components. Two different forms of touch sensibility are recognized: (1) *Simple touch* is concerned with the sense of light touch, light pressure, and a crude sense of tactile localization. Tickling sensation should also be included in this category, but itching is more clearly related to pain sense. (2) *Tactile discrimination* conveys the sense of deeper pressure, spatial localization, and the perception of the size and shape of objects. At least three different spinal cord pathways mediate tactile sensations: (1) the *fasciculi gracilis* and *cuneatus* (discussed in Chapter 6), (2) the *anterior spinothalamic tract* which, along with the lateral spinothalamic tract, comprises the *anterolateral system* (discussed in Chapter 5), and (3) the *lateral cervical system (spinocervicothalamic pathway)*.

THE PATHWAY OF SIMPLE TOUCH

The peripheral receptors are free nerve endings, tactile corpuscles in the dermis of the skin, and networks of nerve terminals around hair follicles. The myelinated fibers which convey sensory impulses from these endings enter the spinal cord by way of dorsal roots. These fibers eventually make synapses in both the posterior and anterior gray horns (laminae VI, VII, VIII), but they do not do so until a considerable amount of longitudinal dispersion has taken place. Some branches of the entering root fibers reach the posterior gray matter within one or two segments. Other branches may extend 10 to 15 segments upward in the posterior funiculi before synapsing in the gray matter of the spinal cord. The second order fibers of the pathway arise from cells of the posterior gray horn, cross in the anterior white commissure and turn upward in anterolateral system as the anterior spinothalamic tract of the opposite side (Fig. 13). The anterior spinothalamic tract, smaller and somewhat more diffuse than the lateral spinothalamic tract, is located near the periphery of the

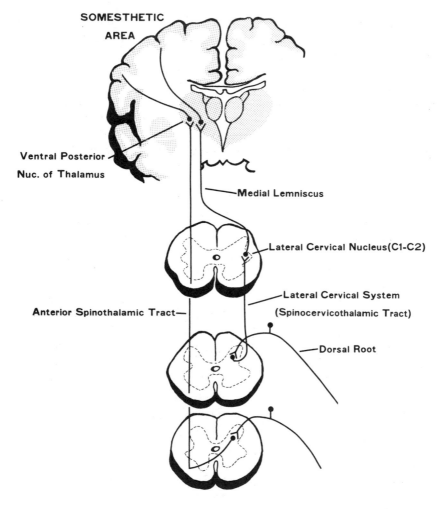

SOMESTHETIC AREA

Ventral Posterior Nuc. of Thalamus

Medial Lemniscus

Lateral Cervical Nucleus(C1-C2)

Lateral Cervical System (Spinocervicothalamic Tract)

Anterior Spinothalamic Tract

Dorsal Root

TACTILE PATHWAYS

FIGURE 13. This diagram depicts two of the three spinal cord pathways that conduct tactile sensations to a conscious level. The third system (posterior column pathways) is diagramed in Figure 12.

37

anterior funiculus. It takes a direct, upward course through the spinal cord and brain stem and most likely terminates in the same structures that receive fibers from the lateral spinothalamic system (see Chapter 5). Thalamocortical fibers relay sensory impulses to the primary and secondary somatic sensory areas of the cerebrum.

Effect of Cutting the Anterior Spinothalamic Tract

Of all types of skin sensibility, simple touch is least likely to be impaired by lesions of the spinal cord. It is not abolished by destruction of the anterior spinothalamic tract on one side, because such information is conveyed through several pathways.

The routine method of testing simple touch is by stroking the skin with a wisp of cotton. This is sufficient for ordinary purposes, but it does not bring out partial loss of sensibility. Von Frey hairs are used for experimental work. These are a series of fine hairs of graduated stiffness for applying stimuli of calibrated intensity to the skin.

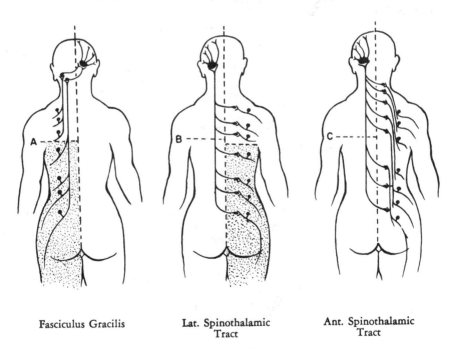

Fasciculus Gracilis   Lat. Spinothalamic Tract   Ant. Spinothalamic Tract

FIGURE 14. Shaded regions show body areas affected by interrupting sensory paths at the midthoracic level of the spinal cord: A. Section of the posterior funiculus (left). B. Section of the lateral spinothalamic tract (left). C. Section of the anterior spinothalamic tract (left).

The Lateral Cervical System

Fibers that convey tactile information synapse in the posterior horn (laminae III and IV) throughout the length of the spinal cord. Heavily myelinated second order neurons arise from these laminae and project ipsilaterally in the posterior aspect of the lateral funiculus and course rostrally to synapse in the *lateral cervical nucleus*, located at C1 and C2 levels. This pathway is called the *spinocervical tract or lateral cervical system* (Fig. 14). Third order fibers from the lateral cervical nucleus cross to the opposite side through the anterior white commissure and join the medial lemniscus at the level of the medulla to project to the thalamus. The entire system, the spinocervicothalamic system, is a very rapidly conducting pathway.

8
Lesions of Nerves and Spinal Cord

Flaccid Paralysis of Muscles – Lower Motor Neuronal Lesion

Destruction of anterior horn cells, ventral nerve roots, or motor fibers of peripheral nerves abolishes both the voluntary and the reflex responses of muscles (see Fig. 9, lesion 2). Besides paralysis, the affected muscles display no tonus and no tendon reflexes can be elicited. Within a few weeks the fibers of these muscles begin to show *atrophy*. The atrophy of muscle fibers deprived of their motor neurons is more profound than the atrophy which occurs in muscles that are rendered inactive. Apparently, the motor horn cell exerts a trophic influence on muscle fibers that is essential for maintaining their normal state. Muscles that are undergoing early stages of atrophy display fibrillary tremors and fasciculations. *Fibrillations* are fine twitchings of single muscle fibers, rarely visible except on the surface of exposed muscle. Fasciculations are brief contractions of a large group of fibers which can be seen through the intact skin.

Lesions which damage fibers of the dorsal roots, or their cell bodies in spinal ganglia, also disrupt the stretch reflex path and, as a consequence, produce hypotonus and loss of tendon reflexes in muscles. In this instance, the lower motor neurons remain intact and there is no loss of voluntary motor strength. The trophic influence of anterior horn cells is not impaired, and muscle atrophy (except that of disuse), or fasciculations do not appear.

Spastic Paralysis of Muscles – Upper Motor Neuronal Lesion

A lesion in the posterior limb of the internal capsule (see Fig. 9, lesion 1) can disrupt the influence of the cerebral cortex upon the contralateral anterior horn cells. The corticospinal tract is only one of many pathways involved in such a lesion. Polysynaptic cortico-rubrospinal and corticoreticulospinal systems are also disrupted. These systems, in turn, are influenced by the basal ganglia and cerebellum. Significantly, the internal capsule lesion could disrupt feedback loops between the cerebrum and cerebellum and between the cerebrum and basal ganglia. Immediately following such a lesion, the stretch reflexes are depressed temporarily, and the paralyzed muscles are flaccid. After an interval, which varies from a few days to a few weeks, stretch reflexes return in these muscles; furthermore, they usually become more active than normal. Increased tonus is demonstrated by firmness and stiffness, especially in the flexor muscles of the arm and the extensors of the leg. Muscle resistance to passive movements is exaggerated. This resistance is strong at the beginning of the movement but gives way in a peculiar *clasp-knife* fashion as more force is applied. Tendon reflexes are hyperactive. Occasionally a quick stretch of a tendon produces *clonus*, a sustained series of rhythmic jerks, instead of a single contraction. Muscles that present these signs of hyperreflexia are said to be *spastic*, or to show *spasticity*. Other conditions may produce hypertonic muscles, but they have distinguishing features which differentiate them from the spasticity associated with internal capsule lesions. Some examples of these are decerebrate rigidity, reflex rigidity, catatonic rigidity, and myotonia.

A discussion of an internal capsule lesion may seem quite out of place in a chapter concerning lesions of nerves and the spinal cord. However, even in view of opposing evidence, it is still taught that all of the symptoms listed in the preceding paragraph occur as a result of a lesion of the corticospinal (pyramidal) tract. Because of this, the disorder has been termed *the classical pyramidal tract syndrome* (that is, spastic paralysis, increased deep tendon reflexes (DTRs), Babinski sign, clasp-knife response to passive movements, clonus, and lack of muscle atrophy except in chronic cases in which disuse atrophy may occur). The corticospinal tract, through its terminal fibers on lower motor neurons, was formerly thought to have the capacity of restricting the activity of the stretch reflex. Spasticity, consequently, was explained as the release of stretch reflexes from the inhibitory influence of the corticospinal tract. It is now known that the activity of this reflex is regulated by the balanced effects of all the fiber tracts which descend to the spinal cord from the brain stem. Some of these fibers have suppressor effects, others are facilitatory. Spasticity and increased deep tendon reflexes are primarily due to reduction of inhibitory influences upon gamma motor neu-

41

rons. The hypersensitive gamma fibers stimulate muscle spindles to a higher rate of discharge, hence increased DTRs and spasticity.

Throughout this book remember that the symptoms listed for corticospinal tract lesions occur because other descending pathways are also usually involved. A pure corticospinal tract lesion below the level of the pyramidal decussation would give rise only to distal flexor muscle weakness and, for unexplained reasons, a Babinski sign on the ipsilateral side. The deficits would occur contralaterally if the lesion were located rostral to the decussation. An isolated lesion of the corticospinal tract rarely occurs clinically.

The effects of lower motor neuron lesions are limited to the muscles that they innervate, but a small lesion that interrupts the corticospinal tract removes voluntary motor control from the whole sector of the body that lies downstream from the level of injury. Thus, destruction of the corticospinal tract in the upper cervical region of the spinal cord paralyzes the arm and the leg on the side of the lesion. If a similar lesion occurs at a site above the decussation of the tract, the paralysis will be in the arm and leg of the opposite side. Paralysis of this sort which includes both the arm and leg is termed *hemiplegia*. *Paraplegia* is paralysis of both legs as, for example, after a transverse lesion of the spinal cord that destroys both pyramidal tracts. Paralysis of a single extremity is *monoplegia*; one that includes all four extremities is *quadriplegia*. Lesions that impair function, but are not severe enough to cause total paralysis produce weakness which is clinically designated as *paresis*.

Other Reflexes Associated with Lesions of the Motor Pathway

Certain reflexes which are not elicited in normal individuals may be present after injuries of the corticospinal tract. Babinski's sign is an abnormal reflex obtained by stroking the plantar surface of the outer border of the foot with a blunt point. The normal response is plantar flexion of the toes, but if Babinski's sign is present, there is a slow dorsiflexion of the great toe accompanied by fanning of the lateral toes. When it is found, Babinski's sign is strong indication of a disorder of the pyramidal system. Many similar pathological reflexes have been described. Hoffmann's sign is sought by flicking the nail of the patient's middle finger. When the sign is present, there is prompt adduction of the thumb and flexion of the index finger. Hoffman's sign is commonly associated with injury of the pyramidal tract, but it is also seen occasionally in normal persons.

Superficial reflexes which are normally obtained by stroking certain areas of the skin may be absent if the corticospinal tract is injured. If the skin of the abdominal wall is scratched gently, the umbilicus normally retracts in the direction of the stimulus. Stroking the upper, inner aspect of the thigh normally causes reflex contraction of the cremaster muscle with elevation of the testicle on the stimulated side. Loss of the *abdominal* or *cremasteric* reflexes confirms the presence of a corticospinal tract lesion, but absence of these reflexes bilaterally in an otherwise normal individual may have no significance.

Lesions of Peripheral Nerves

Injury of an individual peripheral nerve is followed by paralysis of muscles and loss of sensation limited to those muscles and skin areas supplied by the nerve distal to the lesion. The paralyzed muscles are flaccid and gradually undergo severe atrophy. All forms of sensation including proprioception are lost. Recognition of peripheral nerve lesions is based on knowledge of the gross anatomy of the course and distribution of such nerves.

In *multiple neuritis* there is partial destruction of various peripheral nerves. The distribution of the lesions is frequently bilateral, but there may be involvement of nerves in scattered locations. The effects are usually more prominent in the distal parts of the extremities. Muscular weakness and atrophy accompanied by poorly demarked skin areas of sensory changes are characteristic of this disorder.

Lesions of the Posterior Roots

Tabes dorsalis is a form of neurosyphilis which causes bilateral degeneration of dorsal nerve roots and of the posterior funiculi secondarily, particularly in the lower segments of the spinal cord. The paresthesias and intermittent attacks of sharp pain which characteristically appear early in the course of the disease are due to irritation of root fibers. As destruction progresses, there is diminished sensitivity to pain, especially about the tendo achillis and in the testicles. Interruption of the stretch reflex arcs in the posterior roots leads to a loss of the patellar reflexes and ankle jerks. There is severe impairment of muscle sense and vibratory sense. A positive Romberg sign is present. The patient walks with the legs apart, head bend forward, eyes fixed on the ground, throwing the legs excessively high, and slapping the feet down.

Lesions of the Anterior Horns

Acute poliomyelitis, or infantile paralysis, is caused by a virus which selects anterior horn cells, particularly in the cervical and lumbar enlargements of the spinal cord, often damaging them in large numbers. The extent of the muscle paralysis and the muscle groups affected varies, depending on the distribution of motor cells which fail to recover. Paralyzed muscles are flaccid and their reflexes are usually absent. Atrophy develops after several weeks, and paralyzed muscles may ultimately be entirely replaced by connective and adipose tissue. Severe paralysis is likely to result in extensive deformities.

Lesions of the Central Gray Matter

In *syringomyelia* there is softening and cavitation around or near the central canal of the spinal cord, most commonly in the region of the cervical enlargement. A lesion in this position interrupts the lateral spinothalamic fibers which pass ventral to the central canal as they cross from one side to the other. Since these fibers conduct pain and temperature impulses from dermatomes on both sides of the body, the result is loss of pain and temperature sensibility with segmental distribution in the upper extremities on both sides. The spinothalamic tracts themselves remain intact, so there is no sensory impairment in the lower extremities. Proprioception and the sense of simple touch are spared in the affected dermatomes of the arms. A condition such as this in which one type of skin sense is lost and others preserved is referred to as *sensory dissociation.* In later stages of the disease, degeneration often extends to the anterior gray horns and causes paralysis with atrophy of muscles innervated by the segments which are involved. Signs of pyramidal tract damage may appear in the lower extremities as a result of compression by the cystic cavity.

Lesions Involving Both the Anterior Horns and the Pyramidal Tracts

Amyotrophic lateral sclerosis is a fatal disease characterized by destruction of motor cells in the anterior gray horns of the spinal cord together with degeneration of the pyramidal tracts bilaterally. Sensory changes are usually not found. There is weakness and atrophy of

44

some muscles, with spasticity and hyperreflexia in others. The effects may be somewhat irregular in distribution, depending on individual variations in the pattern of the lesions in the spinal cord. The classical form of this disease starts with weakness, atrophy, and fasciculations of the muscles of the hands and arms, followed later by spastic paralysis of the legs. Motor nuclei of cranial nerves in some cases undergo degeneration.

Lesions Involving Posterior and Lateral Funiculi

Subacute combined degeneration is a disease of the spinal cord most often seen in pernicious anemia but sometimes occurring with other types of anemia or nutritional disturbances. The posterior funiculi and the pyramidal tracts of the spinal cord undergo degeneration, but the gray matter is ordinarily not affected. Injury of the posterior funiculi is accompanied by loss of position sense in the lower extremities, impairment of ability to recognize vibration over the legs, and a positive Romberg sign. Motor weakness in the legs, with spasticity, hyperactive tendon reflexes, and bilateral Babinski signs, indicate degeneration of the pyramidal tracts.

Thrombosis of the Anterior Spinal Artery

The anterior spinal artery runs in the anterior median sulcus and sends terminal branches to supply the ventral and lateral portions of the spinal cord. The anterior horns, the lateral spinothalamic tracts, and the pyramidal tracts are included in its territory, but the posterior funiculi and posterior horns are supplied independently by a pair of posterior spinal arteries. Thrombosis of the anterior spinal artery in the cervical region of the cord produces atrophy, fibrillation, and flaccid paralysis at the level of the lesion due to destruction of anterior horn cells. There will also be spastic paraplegia from pyramidal tract involvement and, usually, loss of pain and temperature sense below the lesion due to lateral spinothalamic damage. The onset of symptoms is abrupt and is often accompanied by severe pain.

Hemisection of the Spinal Cord

Lateral hemisection of the spinal cord (as, for example, from a bullet or knife wound) produces the *Brown-Séquard syndrome.* The specific effects and the injured structures that account for them are summarized as follows:

From Injury to Fiber Tracts

I. On the side of the lesion:
   A. Pyramidal tract damage: motor paralysis below the injury with spasticity, hyperactivity reflexes, loss of superficial reflexes, and Babinski's sign.
   B. Posterior funiculus damage: loss of muscle and position sense; loss of vibratory sense and tactile discrimination below the injury. Because of the paralysis, ataxia which might otherwise occur cannot be readily demonstrated.
II. On the side opposite the lesion:
   A. Anterolateral system damage: loss of sensation of pain and temperature beginning one or two dermatomes below the injury.

From Injury to Local Cord Segments and Nerve Roots

Besides the effects produced by interrupting the long ascending and descending tracts of the spinal cord, there are likely to be additional symptoms from damage to dorsal and ventral nerve roots at the level of the injury. When these are present, they are of great value in localizing the individual cord segments involved.
I. On the side of the lesion:
   A. Irritation of fibers in the dorsal root zone: parethesias, or radicular pain in a band over the affected dermatomes.
   B. Destruction of dorsal roots: a band of anesthesia over the dermatome supplied by the involved roots.
   C. Destruction of ventral roots: flaccid paralysis affecting only those muscles innervated by fibers which have been destroyed.
Few lesions are precisely localized to one lateral half of the spinal cord. More often they involve one sector of the cord and produce a partial, or incomplete Brown-Séquard syndrome. The particular symptoms and signs of each individual case are determined by the position and extent of the lesion.

Tumors of the Spinal Cord

Tumors that arise outside the spinal cord (extramedullary tumors) gradually impinge on the cord as they enlarge. Compression of nerve

46

roots is likely to occur first and is responsible for pain distributed over the dermatomes supplied by these roots. This is followed by gradual involvement of the tracts within the spinal cord until a Brown-Séquard syndrome, or some modification of it, is reached. The order of appearance of symptoms may furnish a clue to the site of the tumor. For example, loss of pain and temperature on the left side followed by spastic paralysis on the right implies that the tumor has arisen from the ventrolateral region of the cord on the right side. Loss of proprioception sense on the right side followed by an extension of proprioceptive deficit to the left side and the development of spastic paralysis on the right, indicates that the tumor is compressing the spinal cord from the dorsomedial region on the right side.

Injuries to nerve fibers vary in degree. Some are sufficient to prevent conduction of nerve impulses without causing irreversible fiber degeneration. The pressure of tumors, intervertebral discs, blood clots, or the swelling and edema of wounds may produce spinal cord symptoms that are later alleviated by treatment. The prospect of recovery depends on the pressure and its duration.

Degenerative Changes in Nerve Cells

When a fiber is transected or permanently destroyed, the part which has been separated from the nerve cell body degenerates completely, and in the process, loses its myelin sheath. Degenerated fibers can be studied histologically by obtaining a series of microscopic sections, staining them appropriately, and reconstructing the course of the fibers. The Weigert and Weil methods employ a modified hematoxylin stain which stains normal myelin dark blue or black. An unstained area appearing in the position normally occupied by a fiber tract indicates degeneration. The Marchi method utilizes impregnation of the sections with osmium tetroxide to blacken degenerating nerve fibers while leaving normal myelinated fibers unstained. The test is effective only if osmium tetroxide is applied at a particular stage of the degenerative process when myelin is partly, but not completely, chemically decomposed (generally 6 to 12 days after injury). For this reason the Marchi method is rarely suitable for use with human postmortem material but has been used extensively in experimental work. *The Nauta method and its modifications, (Nauta-Gygax and Fink-Heimer)* are invaluable techniques in tracing degenerating axons. These silver nitrate impregnation techniques have a tremendous advantage over the Marchi method in that the degenerating axon (including its terminal processes, telodendria, and boutons) rather than the myelin sheath is impregnated. Figure 15

47

shows the principal ascending and descending tracts of the spinal cord as they appear in cross section above and below a hemisection after they have been stained to show degenerating fibers.

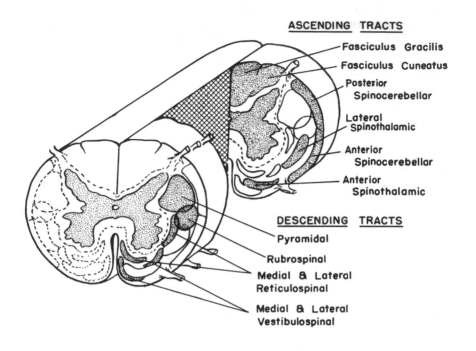

FIGURE 15. Principal tracts of the spinal cord. The descending tracts are shown in the lower cross section; ascending tracts in the upper section. Shaded areas correspond to the regions of degeneration above and below a hemisection of the cord.

Besides causing permanent destruction of the disconnected portion, severing a cell's axon has a harmful effect on the nerve cell body itself. For several weeks after the injury, the Nissl bodies (chromophilic substance) of the cell undergo *chromatolysis*—a process in which extranuclear granules of RNA lose their staining characteristics and seem to dissolve in the surrounding cytoplasm. Some of the affected cells disintegrate, but others recover with restoration of Nissl substance. As Nissl himself realized, this retrograde chromatolytic reaction furnishes a means of determining the cells of origin for fibers. Some weeks following an experimental lesion, serial sections can be made and stained for Nissl substance with a basic aniline dye. A careful search may then reveal specific areas of chromatolysis.

Regeneration of Nerve Fibers

A completely severed peripheral nerve has some capacity to repair itself. *Schwann* (neurolemma) cells from the isolated stump proliferate and attempt to bridge the gap with the distal end of the nerve. The axis cylinders in the cut, in the central end of the nerve divide longitudinally and soon begin to sprout out of the end of the nerve. Many sprouting axons go astray in random directions, but some of them cross the gap and enter neurilemmal tubes leading to the peripheral endings. Their rate of growth is normally 1 to 2 mm per day. Chance apparently determines whether a regenerating motor fiber enters a neurilemmal tube leading to a motor or to a sensory terminal. If suitably matched, connections with a motor end-plate can be reestablished and function restored. Fibers of the brain and of the spinal cord, however, do not regenerate effectively.

9
Brain Stem

The brain stem is divided into the medulla, pons, midbrain, and diencephalon.

MEDULLA

The medulla (medulla oblongata) (bulb) is continuous with the spinal cord at the foramen magnum and extends 2.5 cm to the caudal border of the pons. The central canal of the spinal cord continues through the caudal half of the medulla, and then, at a point called the *obex*, flares open into the wide cavity of the *fourth ventricle* posteriorly. The posterior surface of the upper half of the medulla thus occupies the lateral floor of the ventricle. The roof of this part of the medulla is formed by the *chorioid plexus*, a thin sheet of ependyma and pia mater.

External Markings of the Medulla

ANTERIOR (VENTRAL) ASPECT (Fig. 16). The *pyramids*, which contain the pyramidal (corticospinal) tracts, form two longitudinal ridges on either side of the anterior median fissure. Their decussation can be seen obliterating the fissure at the extreme caudal end of the medulla.

LATERAL ASPECT (Fig. 17). Two longitudinal grooves are present. The anterolateral sulcus extends along the lateral border of the pyramid and contains the row of rootlets of the hypoglossal nerve (n.

50

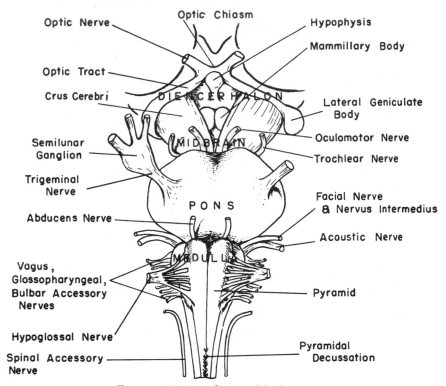

Optic Nerve

Optic Chiasm

Hypophysis

Mammillary Body

Optic Tract

Crus Cerebri

DIENCEPHALON

Lateral Geniculate Body

Semilunar Ganglion

MIDBRAIN

Oculomotor Nerve

Trochlear Nerve

Trigeminal Nerve

PONS

Facial Nerve & Nervus Intermedius

Abducens Nerve

Acoustic Nerve

Vagus, Glossopharyngeal, Bulbar Accessory Nerves

MEDULLA

Hypoglossal Nerve

Pyramid

Spinal Accessory Nerve

Pyramidal Decussation

FIGURE 16. Ventral view of the brain stem.

XII). Radicles of the accessory nerve (n. XI), vagus nerve (n. X), and glossopharyngeal nerve (n. IX) are attached in line along the posterolateral sulcus. The prominent oval swelling of the lateral area between these sulci is the *olive*. This marks the site of the inferior olivary nuclear complex inside the medulla.

POSTERIOR (DORSAL) ASPECT (Fig. 18). The fasciculus gracilis and the fasciculus cuneatus are visible as low ridges. The sites of the nucleus gracilis and the nucleus cuneatus are marked by small eminences named, respectively, the *clava* and the *cuneate tubercle*. Rostral to the obex, separation of the left and right posterior plates of the medulla exposes the floor of the fourth ventricle. The two prominent ridges extending along the sides of the ventricle are the *inferior cerebellar peduncles* (restiform bodies). Two pairs of small swellings can be seen in the floor of the ventricle. Their tapering margins point caudally and gradually meet the groove of the medial sulcus in a configuration named the *calamus scriptorius* from its resemblance to the point of a pen. The lateral ridges of the calamus constitute the *vagal trigone*; the medial ridges are the *hypoglossal trigone*. Rostral

51

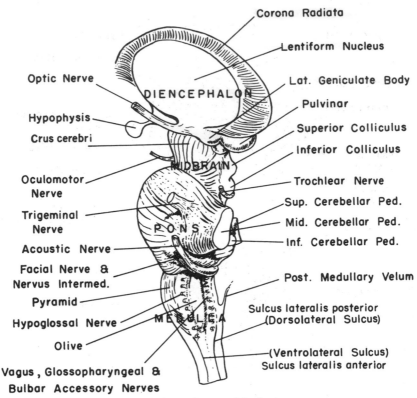

Optic Nerve

Hypophysis

Crus cerebri

Oculomotor
Nerve

Trigeminal
Nerve

Acoustic Nerve

Facial Nerve &
Nervus Intermed.

Pyramid

Hypoglossal Nerve

Olive

Vagus, Glossopharyngeal &
Bulbar Accessory Nerves

Corona Radiata

Lentiform Nucleus

Lat. Geniculate Body

Pulvinar

Superior Colliculus

Inferior Colliculus

Trochlear Nerve

Sup. Cerebellar Ped.

Mid. Cerebellar Ped.

Inf. Cerebellar Ped.

Post. Medullary Velum

Sulcus lateralis posterior
(Dorsolateral Sulcus)

(Ventrolateral Sulcus)
Sulcus lateralis anterior

DIENCEPHALON

MIDBRAIN

PONS

MEDULLA

FIGURE 17. Lateral view of the brain stem.

to the *stria of the fourth ventricle* is the *facial colliculus*. The rostral continuation of the ridge is known as the *medial eminence*. The groove on the lateral margin of these central ridges is the *sulcus limitans* which demarcates the sensory and motor areas of the medulla.

Internal Structures of the Medulla

Some of the long fiber tracts of the spinal cord pass directly through the medulla without any major changes in their relative positions, but otherwise the arrangement of fibers and gray substance of the medulla is more complex than in the spinal cord.

CAUDAL HALF OF THE MEDULLA (Figs. 19 and 20). The central canal is surrounded by a *central gray area* which is modified at its perimeter to become a diffuse zone containing a network of fibers and scattered cells known as the *reticular formation*. The reticular formation extends through the medulla, pons, and mesencephalon.

52

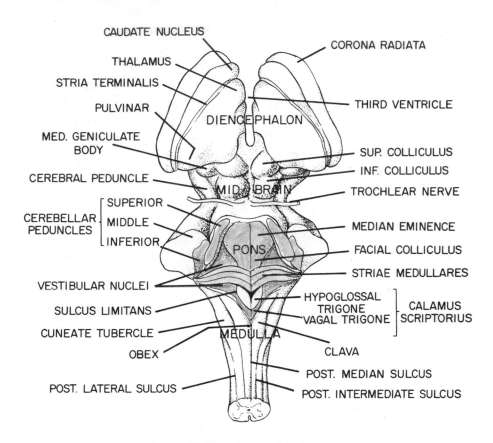

FIGURE 18. Dorsal view of the brain stem.

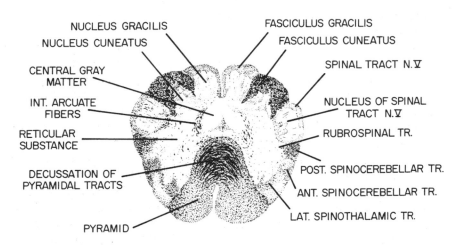

FIGURE 19. Cross section of the extreme lower region of the medulla.

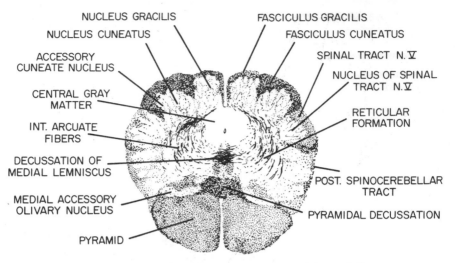

NUCLEUS GRACILIS
NUCLEUS CUNEATUS
ACCESSORY
CUNEATE NUCLEUS
CENTRAL GRAY
MATTER
INT. ARCUATE
FIBERS
DECUSSATION OF
MEDIAL LEMNISCUS
MEDIAL ACCESSORY
OLIVARY NUCLEUS
PYRAMID

FASCICULUS GRACILIS
FASCICULUS CUNEATUS
SPINAL TRACT N. V
NUCLEUS OF SPINAL
TRACT N. V
RETICULAR
FORMATION
POST. SPINOCEREBELLAR
TRACT
PYRAMIDAL DECUSSATION

FIGURE 20. Cross section of the lower region of the medulla.

The *corticospinal tracts* occupy the most anterior part of the medulla and, at this point, cross in a prominent *decussation* which brings them to the lateral position that they maintain in the spinal cord. On the posterior side the *fasciculi gracilis and cuneatus* are still present, but the nuclei in which their fibers terminate have appeared. Axons of the cells in these nuclei take a downward, arched course forming the *internal arcuate fibers* which cross the midline as the *decussation of the medial lemniscus*. In the posterolateral region a clear nuclear area, capped by a peripheral zone of fine fibers, represents the *spinal tract and spinal nucleus of the trigeminal nerve*. The latter structures remain in the same relative position as they descend from the pontine region.

ROSTRAL HALF OF THE MEDULLA (Fig. 21). The *inferior olivary nuclear complex* is a prominent structure in the anterolateral region resembling a crinkled sac with an opening directed toward the midline. Many of its efferent fibers cross and stream toward the posterolateral corner of the medulla to join spinocerebellar fibers in the thick, *inferior cerebellar peduncle*. Other olivocerebellar fibers enter the peduncle without crossing.

Three distinct cellular areas (symmetrically paired) occupy the posterior part of the medulla close to the floor of the ventricle. Since they extend longitudinally through the upper medulla, they represent three nuclear columns. The *nucleus of the hypoglossal nerve* (n. XII) is nearest the midline. Fibers of this nerve pass anteriorly to emerge between the pyramid and the olive. The *dorsal motor nucleus* of the vagus nerve (n. X) lies at the side of the hypoglossal

54

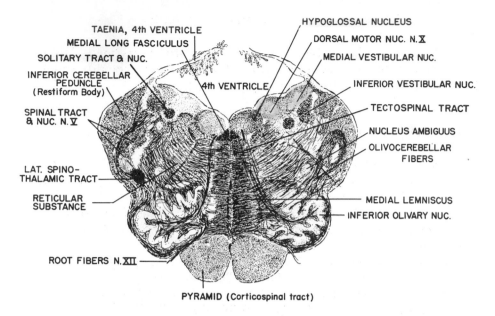

FIGURE 21 Cross section of the upper region of the medulla.

nucleus. The most lateral nuclear column, demarcated by the sulcus limitans, contains the medial and spinal, or inferior *vestibular nuclei* which receive afferent fibers from the vestibular division of the acoustic nerve (n. VIII).

The *nucleus ambiguus,* seen indistinctly in Weigert stained preparations, is located in the anterolateral part of the reticular formation. Its fibers are directed posteromedially at first, but they arch back and leave the medulla anterior to the inferior cerebellar peduncle along with other fibers of the vagus nerve. An isolated bundle of longitudinal fibers accompanied by a small nucleus appears in the posterior part of the reticular formation. It is known as the *solitary tract* and is made up of afferent root fibers of the vagal system. The *nucleus of the solitary tract* lies beside it.

The anterolateral system is adjacent to the nucleus ambiguus on its anterolateral side. Two large bands of fibers lie vertically at either side of the midline. The extreme posterior position of each band contains the *medial longitudinal fasciculus (MLF),* a structure that extends from the upper cervical segment to the midbrain. At this level in the medulla it contains several descending pathways, including the *medial vestibulospinal, tectospinal, interstitiospinal,* and *pontine reticulospinal tracts.* The *medial lemiscus* comprises the remainder and largest portion of this vertical band.

55

PONS

The pons is a large oblong-shaped mass rostral to the medulla. The cerebral peduncles pass into it from above, and the pyramids emerge from its caudal margin.

External Markings of the Pons

ANTERIOR ASPECT (see Fig. 16). The surface is entirely occupied by a band of thick transverse fibers which constitutes the pons proper. A shallow furrow (the basal sulcus) extends along the midline coinciding with the course of the basilar artery. The *abducens nerves* (n. VI) take exit in the inferior pontine sulcus at the caudal border of the pons close to the pyramids.

LATERAL ASPECT (see Fig. 17). The transverse fibers of the pons are funnelled into compact lateral bundles—the *middle cerebellar peduncles* (brachia pontis)—which attach the pons to the overlying cerebellum. The triangular space formed between the caudal border of the middle cerebellar peduncle, the adjoining part of the cerebellum, and the upper part of the medulla constitute the *pontocerebellar angle*. The *facial nerve* (n. VII) and the *acoustic nerve* (n. VIII) are attached to the brain stem in this niche. The *trigeminal nerve* (n. V), one of the largest of the cranial nerves, penetrates the brachium pontis near the middle of the lateral surface of the pons.

POSTERIOR ASPECT (see Fig. 18). The posterior surface of the pons forms the rostral floor of the fourth ventricle. It is a triangular area with its widest point at the pontomedullary junction where the lateral recesses of the ventricle are situated. Faint transverse striations observed in this region are named the *striae medullares* which are really formed by arcuatocerebellar fibers totally unrelated to the acoustic system. The two bands which course along the sides of the triangular space are the *superior cerebellar peduncles* (brachia conjunctiva). The *anterior medullary velum* is a thin layer of tissue completing the roof of the ventricle.

Internal Structure of the Pons

Two subdivisions are evident—a posterior portion known as the *tegmentum,* and an anterior part called the *basilar portion* of the pons. In this region of the brain stem, the roof portion, overlying the cavity of the ventricle, has become expanded and specialized to form the cerebellum.

CAUDAL PORTION (Fig. 22). The corticospinal tracts are located centrally in the basilar portion. The gray matter which surrounds them contains the cells of the *pontine nuclei.* Transverse fibers (pontocerebellar tract) crossing from one side to the other posterior and anterior to the corticospinal tracts are the axons of the pontine nuclei. They enter the *middle cerebellar peduncle* and pass to the cortex of the cerebellum.

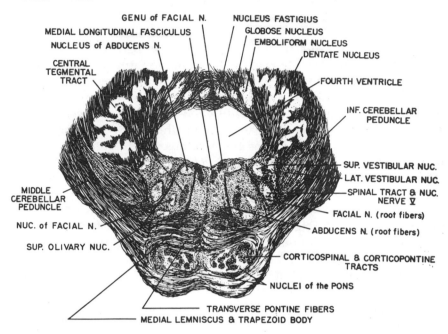

GENU of FACIAL N.
MEDIAL LONGITUDINAL FASCICULUS
NUCLEUS of ABDUCENS N.
CENTRAL TEGMENTAL TRACT
NUCLEUS FASTIGIUS
GLOBOSE NUCLEUS
EMBOLIFORM NUCLEUS
DENTATE NUCLEUS
FOURTH VENTRICLE
INF. CEREBELLAR PEDUNCLE
SUP. VESTIBULAR NUC.
LAT. VESTIBULAR NUC.
SPINAL TRACT & NUC. NERVE Ⅴ
FACIAL N. (root fibers)
ABDUCENS N. (root fibers)
CORTICOSPINAL & CORTICOPONTINE TRACTS
NUCLEI of the PONS
MIDDLE CEREBELLAR PEDUNCLE
NUC. of FACIAL N.
SUP. OLIVARY NUC.
TRANSVERSE PONTINE FIBERS
MEDIAL LEMNISCUS & TRAPEZOID BODY

FIGURE 22. Cross section of the lower region of the pons.

The *medial lemniscus* is seen as an ellipsoid mass extending transversely in contact with the basilar portion of the pons. The *medial longitudinal fasciculus* retains its position near the midline in the floor of the fourth ventricle. At this level, the main ascending fibers in this fasciculus arise from the vestibular nuclei and project primarily to the nuclei supplying the extraocular muscles. The *interstitiospinal, pontine reticulospinal, tectospinal,* and *tectobulbar tracts* are partially intermingled with the MLF.

The *trapezoid body* (an auditory relay structure) is a prominent band of decussating fibers intermingled with small nuclear groups in the anterior part of the tegmentum. Its fibers interlace at right angles with those of the medial lemniscus. The *superior olive* is a small oval nucleus which lies lateral and slightly posterior to the trapezoid body. The *central tegmental tract* is an isolated bundle in the anterior part of the reticular formation containing descending pathways (*cortico-olivary* and *rubro-olivary tracts*) and part of a very important ascending projection, the *ascending reticular activating system* which projects primarily to the *thalamus* and *hypothalamus*. The nucleus and spinal root of the trigeminal nerve have not changed their position, but they now are covered on the lateral side by the inferior and middle cerebellar peduncles.

Immediately posterior to the superior olive, and medial to the nucleus of the spinal root of the trigeminal nerve (n. V) is the pear-shaped *motor nucleus of the facial nerve* (n. VII). Before leaving the brain stem, the fibers of the facial nerve form an internal loop (*the internal genu of the facial nerve*). The first leg of this loop courses posteromedially toward the floor of the fourth ventricle passing close to, and just caudal to, the *nucleus of the abducens nerve*. The facial nerve circles medially around the abducens nucleus returning on the rostral side of the nucleus. After completing this hairpin bend, the nerve takes a direct course, anterolaterally and slightly caudally to its exit at the pontomedullary junction. Fibers of the abducens nerve take a course similar to those of the hypoglossal, passing close to the lateral border of the pyramidal tract to emerge on the anterior aspect of the brain stem.

Nuclei of the *vestibular group* continue to occupy the lateral area in the floor of the fourth ventricle. The individual subnuclei at this level are the lateral and superior, instead of the medial and spinal (inferior) which are found in the medulla.

Paired cerebellar nuclei are generally observed in sections through the cerebellum in the lower level of the pons (see Fig. 22). The nuclei are:

1. Nucleus fastigii — located in midline of roof of fourth ventricle in the region of the vermis.
2. Nucleus globosus — small group of cells located just lateral to above nucleus.
3. Nucleus emboliformis — slightly elongated cellular mass located between the globose and dentate nuclei.
4. Nucleus dentatus — the largest and most lateral of the cerebellar nuclei. It is similar in appearance to the inferior olivary nuclear complex, purse-like, in shape with an anteromedial hilum.

MIDDLE PORTION (Fig. 23). The basilar portion of the pons is widened and thickened. The corticospinal tracts are now dispersed in separate fascicles. Mingling with them are numerous other scattered longitudinal fibers. These are the *corticopontine tracts* descending from the frontal, temporal, parietal, and occipital lobes to synapse with cells of the pontine nuclei.

Two oval-shaped nuclei lie side by side in the posterolateral part

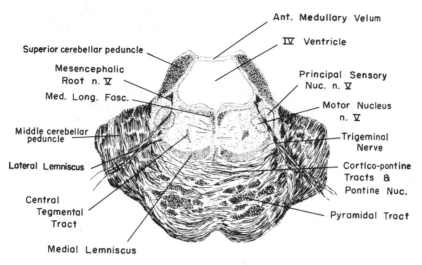

Ant. Medullary Velum

IV Ventricle

Superior cerebellar peduncle

Mesencephalic Root n. V

Med. Long. Fasc.

Principal Sensory Nuc. n. V

Motor Nucleus n. V

Middle cerebellar peduncle

Trigeminal Nerve

Lateral Lemniscus

Cortico-pontine Tracts & Pontine Nuc.

Central Tegmental Tract

Pyramidal Tract

Medial Lemniscus

FIGURE 23. Cross section of the middle region of the pons.

of the tegmentum. The more lateral one is the *principal sensory nuclus of the trigeminal nerve;* the medial is the *motor nucleus (masticator nucleus) of the trigeminal nerve.* Small filaments of the nerve pass posteriorly as the mesencephalic root of the trigeminal nerve. Trigeminal fibers emerging from the surface of the pons pass directly through the middle cerebellar peduncle in an anterolateral direction.

The *superior cerebellar peduncles* (brachia conjunctiva) appear at the sides of the fourth ventricle as large compact bands. The anterior medullary velum forms the roof of the ventricle.

MIDBRAIN

The midbrain is a short segment between the pons and the diencephalon. It is traversed by the *cerebral aqueduct,* an extraordinarily small tubular passage connecting the third ventricle with the fourth.

External Markings of the Midbrain

ANTERIOR ASPECT (see Fig. 16). The inferior surface is formed by two rope-like bundles of fibers, the *crura cerebri,* and a deep *interpeduncular fossa* which separates them. Just before it disappears within the substance of the cerebral hemisphere above, each peduncle is skirted by the optic tract (n. II). At its caudal end, the peduncle passes directly into the basilar portion of the pons. The *oculomotor nerves* (n. III) take exit from the sides of the interpeduncular fossa and emerge on the surface at the transverse groove between the pons and the midbrain.

POSTERIOR ASPECT (see Fig. 18). The posterior surface of the midbrain presents four rounded elevations—the *corpora quadrigemina* (tectum of the midbrain). The rostral pair of swellings are the *superior colliculi;* the somewhat smaller, caudal pair are the *inferior colliculi.* The *trochlear nerves* (n. IV), smallest of the cranial nerves, emerge from the posterior surface just behind the inferior colliculi after decussating in the anterior medullary velum.

Internal Structures of the Midbrain

In cross sections three zones are designated: (1) a basal portion, or crus cerebri, (2) the *tegmentum,* similar to the pontine tegmentum (the crus cerebri and the tegmentum together make up the *cerebral peduncle*), and (3) the *tectum,* or roof portion, lying above the aqueduct and forming the quadrigeminal plate.

CAUDAL HALF OF THE MIDBRAIN (level of the *inferior colliculus*) (Fig. 24). Each crus cerebri appears, in cross section, as a prominent, crescent-shaped mass of fibers within which the corticospinal tract occupies a central position, flanked at either side by corticopontine fibers. A brown-pigmented area of gray matter, known as the *substantia nigra,* lies between the peduncles and the tegmentum.

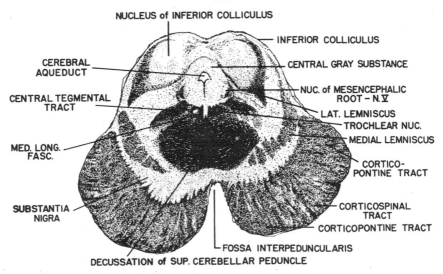

NUCLEUS of INFERIOR COLLICULUS
INFERIOR COLLICULUS
CEREBRAL AQUEDUCT
CENTRAL GRAY SUBSTANCE
NUC. of MESENCEPHALIC ROOT – N.Ⅴ
CENTRAL TEGMENTAL TRACT
LAT. LEMNISCUS
TROCHLEAR NUC.
MEDIAL LEMNISCUS
MED. LONG. FASC.
CORTICO-PONTINE TRACT
SUBSTANTIA NIGRA
CORTICOSPINAL TRACT
CORTICOPONTINE TRACT
FOSSA INTERPEDUNCULARIS
DECUSSATION of SUP. CEREBELLAR PEDUNCLE

FIGURE 24. Cross section of the lower region of the midbrain.

The central part of the tegmentum contains a massive interlace of fibers — *the decussation of the superior cerebellar peduncle.* The *medial lemniscus* is displaced laterally and rotated slightly. Its outer border is in close relation to adjacent fibers of the anterolateral system. The *lateral lemniscus,* containing ascending fibers of the special sensory path of hearing, is clearly defined in the lateral part of the tegmentum posterior to the anterolateral system. The small, globular *nucleus of the trochlear nerve* lies near the *medial longitudinal fasciculus* in the anterior part of the central gray substance. An area of gray matter, the *nucleus of the inferior colliculus,* underlies each colliculus in the tectal region.

ROSTRAL HALF OF THE MIDBRAIN (level of the *superior colliculus*) (Fig. 25). The crura cerebri and the substantia nigra continue to occupy the basal portion.

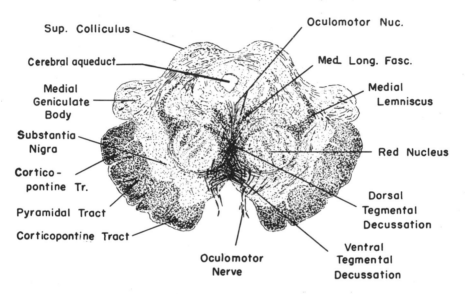

FIGURE 25. Cross section of the upper region of the midbrain.

The *red nuclei* are conspicuous globular masses in the anterior portion of the tegmentum. The crossed fibers of the superior cerebellar peduncle pass into this nucleus and around its edges. Many of them terminate in the red nucleus; others pass forward to the thalamus. The *tectospinal* and *rubrospinal tracts* arise from this part of the midbrain. Both tracts cross near their origin — the tectospinal in the *dorsal tegmental decussation* (fountain decussation of Meynert) and the rubrospinal in the *ventral tegmental decussation* (decussation of Forel).

The nuclear complex of the oculomotor nerve lies in the anterior

61

part of the central gray matter with the *medial longitudinal fasciculus* beside it. The root fibers of the oculomotor nerve stream through and around the red nucleus before converging at their exit in the interpeduncular fossa.

The *medial geniculate bodies* appear as projections on the lateral surfaces of the midbrain. They are auditory-sensory relay centers, properly considered to be a part of the thalamus.

10

Functional Components of the Cranial Nerves

The cranial nerves which have a function similar to that exhibited by the spinal nerves are classified as *general*. The cranial nerves which have specialized functions, such as supplying the eye and ear, conveying the olfactory and gustatory impulses, or innervating the branchiomeric muscles, are classified as *special*.

The above criteria sometimes result in questionable classification. In these cases, custom has precedence and reasons for the choice become apparent.

Résumé of Functional Components

A. General afferent fibers

Sensory fibers which have their cells of origin in the cranio-spinal ganglia.

  1. Somatic afferent (GSA)

     Fibers which carry the exteroceptive (pain, temperature, and touch) and the proprioceptive impulses from sensory endings in the body wall, tendons, and joints.

  2. Visceral afferent (GVA)

     Fibers that carry sensory impulses (generally pain) from the visceral structures within the body.

B. Special afferent fibers

This category is found only in the cranial nerves.

  1. Somatic afferent (SSA)

     Nerves which carry the sensory impulses from the special

63

sense organs, the ear **and the eye** (vision, hearing, and equilibrium).

2. Visceral afferent (SVA)

Fibers which are concerned with the specialized olfactory and gustatory receptors. These fibers are designated as visceral because of the functional association of the sensation with the digestive tract.

C. General efferent fibers

Motor fibers which innervate the musculature of the body (except the branchiomeric fibers).

1. Somatic efferent (GSE)

Fibers which convey the motor impulse to the somatic skeletal muscle (myotomic origin). The bulk of the fibers in the ventral root of the spinal nerve are of this type.

2. Visceral efferent (GVE)

Autonomic fibers which innervate smooth and cardiac muscle fibers and regulate glandular secretion. This category, which may be subdivided into the sympathetic and parasympathetic systems, is found in the spinal nerves and some cranial nerves.

D. Special efferent fibers

Cranial nerves which innervate a specialized area of the skeletal musculature.

1. Visceral efferent (SVE)

Nerve components which innervate striated skeletal muscles derived from the branchial arches. These fibers are not a part of the autonomic nervous system.

THE ANATOMICAL POSITION OF CRANIAL NERVE NUCLEI IN THE BRAIN STEM

The lateral walls of the embryonic brain and spinal cord are demarcated into an alar and a basal lamina by the appearance of the sulcus limitans early in development. The motor nuclei in the basal plate differentiate slightly earlier than the sensory nuclei located in the alar plate. The localization of the various cranial nerve nuclei are indicated and labelled according to their function (Fig. 26).

The general somatic efferent fibers of the cranial nerves III, IV, VI, and XII arise from nuclei which are arranged as a discontinuous column of cells in the floor of the basal plate adjacent to the midline. They are continuous with and homologous to the anterior horn cells. They all innervate musculature derived from somitic myotomes. The general visceral efferent nuclei occupy a position lateral to the so-

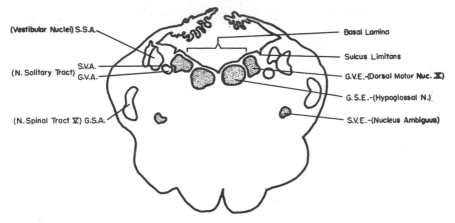

FIGURE 26. Outline cross section of the upper region of the medulla. (Compare with Figure 21.)

matic efferent column. The motor nuclei of cranial nerves V, VII, IX, X, and XI, which provide the innervation of the branchiomeric musculature and are designated as the special visceral efferent nuclei, form the most lateral discontinuous column of neurons derived from the basal lamina.

The sensory fibers terminate in nuclei which are located in the alar lamina. Figure 26 indicates that the special somatic afferent fibers terminate in the most posterior portion of the alar plate. The visceral afferent fibers terminate in a nuclear area adjacent to the visceral efferent column. The nucleus of the tractus solitarius serves as the receptor site — the cephalic portion of the nucleus receives the gustatory fiber terminals. The general somatic afferent column extends from the midbrain to the caudal extent of the medulla. It is subdivided into the mesencephalic nucleus, the principal sensory nucleus, and the nucleus of the spinal tract, all being parts of the trigeminal nerve. It will be noticed that the latter nucleus, that of the spinal tract, is continuous with the substantia gelatinosa and the dorsolateral fasciculus. The later spinal cord and cranial components have the same function — pain and temperature reception.

Upon entrance into the brain stem, the cranial nerves subdivide into a variable number of fibers which make connections with their respective nuclei. For example, the nucleus ambiguus is the site of origin of the special visceral efferent fibers for the IX, X, and the bulbar portion of the XI cranial nerves. Likewise, the central processes of the gustatory fibers of the cranial nerves VII, IX, and X synapse with neurons in the cephalic portion of the nucleus of the tractus solitarius.

65

Functional Components in the Cranial Nerves

1. Olfactory nerve

   Special visceral afferent. The fila from the *bipolar olfactory epithelial cells* constitute the olfactory nerve and they terminate in the olfactory bulb.

2. Optic nerve

   Special somatic afferent. The fibers (third order neurons) which arise from the ganglion cells of the retina constitute the so-called nerve. It is not a true nerve but represents an evaginated fiber tract of the diencephalon. The fibers from the nasal halves of the retina decussate in the optic chiasma.

3. Oculomotor nerve

   General somatic efferent. The fibers arise in the oculomotor nucleus and innervate the extrinsic mucles of the eye — except the superior oblique and the lateral rectus. The muscles arise from preotic myotomes; thus, the term general.

   General visceral efferent. Consists of the preganglionic parasympathetic fibers which arise in the accessory oculomotor (Edinger-Westphal) nucleus and terminate in the ciliary ganglion. They participate in the light and accommodation reflexes.

   General somatic afferent. Consists of the proprioceptive fibers for the extrinsic muscles innervated by the third nerve. These fibers have their cell bodies of origin located in the mesencephalic nucleus of the trigeminal nerve. This is the exception to the general rule that all primary afferents must have their cell bodies located in peripheral ganglia.

4. Trochlear nerve

   General somatic efferent. Fibers arise in the trochlear nucleus and innervate the superior oblique muscle of the eye which is derived from the preotic myotomes.

   General somatic afferent. Consists of the proprioceptive fibers from the superior oblique muscles. Termination is unknown, but may possibly be in the mesencephalic nucleus of the trigeminal nerve.

5. Trigeminal nerve

   General somatic afferent

   Exteroceptive fibers. Sensory fibers from the skin of the face and scalp and the ectodermal mucous membranes of the head (mouth and nasal chamber). The cells of origin are located in the semilunar ganglion.

   Proprioceptive fibers. Sensory fibers from the muscles of mastication and the other muscles innervated by the mandibular nerve. The cells of origin are located in the mesencephalic nucleus of the trigeminal nerve.

Special visceral efferent. Fibers from the motor nucleus of the fifth nerve through the portio minor and mandibular nerve which innervate the muscles of mastication, tensor veli palati, tensor tympani, mylohyoid, and the anterior belly of the digastric. These muscles arise from the first branchial arch.

6. Abducens nerve

General somatic efferent. Fibers which arise in the abducens nucleus innervate the lateral rectus muscle of the eye which is derived from the preotic myotomes.

General somatic afferent. Consists of the proprioceptive fibers from the lateral rectus muscle. Termination is unknown, but probably similar to that of the trochlear nerve.

7. Facial nerve

General somatic afferent. Cell bodies located in the geniculate ganglion have fibers conveying exteroceptive sensations (pain and temperature) from the region of the ear.

General visceral afferent. Fibers have cells of origin in the geniculate ganglion. The peripheral fibers receive the sensations of deep sensibility from the face. The fibers are a component of the nervus intermedius.

Special visceral afferent. Cells of origin in the geniculate ganglion. Peripheral fibers terminate in the taste buds on the anterior two-thirds of the tongue. The fibers reach the tongue by way of the intermediate nerve, chorda tympani, and lingual nerve. Central branches terminate in the rostral portion of the nucleus solitarius.

General visceral efferent. The preganglionic parasympathetic fibers which arise in the superior salivatory nucleus and synapse with the postganglionic neurons in the pterygopalatine and the submandibular ganglia. Preganglionic fibers are a component of the nervus intermedius.

Special visceral efferent. Fibers arise from neurons in the motor nucleus of the seventh nerve. They innervate the superficial muscles of the face and scalp (muscles of facial expression), the platysma, stylohyoid, and the posterior belly of the digastric. These muscles originate from the second arch.

8. Vestibulocochlear (statoacoustic) nerve
Special somatic afferent

Exteroceptive fibers. The cochlear nerve has bipolar cells of origin in the spinal ganglion. Peripheral processes receive stimuli from the hair cells in the cochlear duct. The central processes terminate in the posterior and anterior cochlear nuclei.

Proprioceptive fibers. The vestibular nerve has bipolar cells that originate in the vestibular ganglion. Peripheral processes receive stimuli from hair cells in maculae (of the utricle and saccule) and cristae (in the ampullae of the semicircular canals). The central processes terminate in vestibular nuclei.

9. Glossopharyngeal nerve

General somatic afferent. Cell bodies located in the superior ganglion have fibers conveying exteroceptive sensations (pain and temperature) from the region of the ear.

General visceral afferent. The cell bodies located in the inferior ganglion (petrosal) have peripheral fibers which carry general sensory fibers from the posterior third of the tongue and the pharynx. The central processes terminate in the nucleus of the solitary tract.

Special visceral afferent. The cell bodies of the same ganglion have peripheral fibers which carry the gustatory sense from the posterior third of the tongue. Central processes terminate in the rostral portion of the nucleus of the solitary tract.

General visceral efferent. Preganglionic parasympathetic fibers from cells in the inferior salivatory nucleus terminate in the otic ganglion. Postganglionic fibers of the ganglion innervate the parotid gland.

Special visceral efferent. Fibers originating from neurons in the nucleus ambiguus innervate the skeletal muscle of the third visceral arch (stylopharyngeus).

10. Vagus nerve

General somatic afferent. Cell bodies located in the superior ganglion (jugular) have fibers conveying exteroceptive sensations (pain and temperature) from the region of the ear.

General visceral afferent. Cell bodies located in the inferior ganglion (nodose) have fibers conveying exteroceptive sensations from the pharynx, larynx, thoracic, and abdominal viscera.

Special visceral afferent. Peripheral processes of neurons in the inferior ganglion receive gustatory stimuli from epiglottal taste buds by way of the internal laryngeal nerve.

General visceral efferent. Preganglionic parasymphathetic fibers from neurons in the dorsal motor nucleus of nerve X innervate the thoracic and abdominal viscera of glands, cardiac and smooth muscle to the level of the splenic flexure of the colon. It will be remembered that the postganglionic neurons are located in the visceral walls.

Special visceral efferent. Fibers from cells in the nucleus ambiguus innervate the skeletal musculature of the remaining branchial arches (soft palate, larynx, and pharnyx).

11. Spinal accessory nerve

General somatic afferent. Proprioceptive fibers from the skeletal muscles are innervated by this nerve. The cells of origin, located in the upper cervical spinal ganglia, reach the muscles through branchings of the cervical plexus.

General visceral efferent. The fibers which arise in the dorsal motor nucleus of nerve X to rejoin the vagus nerve. They are believed to form components of the cardiac branches of the vagus nerve.

Special visceral efferent. (1) Fibers arising from neurons in the nucleus ambiguus accompany those of the vagus nerve and supply the skeletal musculature, in part, of the pharynx and larynx. (2) A second group of fibers, which have their origin from neurons in the anterior gray horn of the cervical spinal cord, innervate the sternocleidomastoid and trapezius muscles.

12. Hypoglossal nerve

General somatic efferent. Fibers which arise from neurons in the hypoglossal nucleus and innervate the skeletal musculature of the tongue which is derived from the three occipital myotomes.

General somatic afferent. Proprioceptive fibers from the lingual musculature (similar to that proposed for cranial nerve III, IV, and VI). Scattered neurons, which have been found along the nerve, have been postulated to be the ganglion cells which serve this function.

Note: The nervus terminalis has been omitted from the summary as it has been studied primarily in the lower vertebrates.

11

Cranial Nerves of the Medulla

HYPOGLOSSAL NERVE (NERVE XII)

The hypoglossal nerve is the motor nerve of the tongue muscula-ture. Its general somatic efferent fibers are lower motor neuron fibers originating in cells of the hypoglossal nucleus. Among the muscles supplied by the hypoglossal nerve are the genioglossi which, by their posterior fibers, draw the root of the tongue forward and cause the tip of the tongue to protrude. Hemiparalysis, or hemiparesis, of the tongue results in unbalanced action of the genioglossus muscles. Consequently, on voluntary protrusion, the tongue deviates to the paralyzed side.

ACCESSORY NERVE (NERVE XI)

The accessory nerve has two distinct parts. The spinal root, which arises from anterior horn cells of cervical cord segments (spinal accessory nucleus) one through five, ascends through the foramen magnum and courses along the side of the medulla. Here it joins the bulbar root from the medulla. After accompanying the spinal root fibers for a short distance, the bulbar fibers turn away to join the vagus nerve and are distributed with the terminal branches of the vagus. The spinal portion of nerve XI (special visceral efferent fibers) passes through the jugular foramen and descends in the neck to end in the sternomastoid and trapezius muscles. The spinal division of the accessory is a displaced loop of the cervical plexus and not a true cranial nerve.

70

VAGUS NERVE COMPLEX
(NERVES IX, X, AND PORTIONS OF NERVES VII, XI)

Four nerves of the medulla are closely related in functions and in the configuration of their nuclear groups: (1) the nervus intermedius, the sensory and parasympathetic division of the facial nerve (n. VII); (2) the glossopharyngeal nerve (n. IX); (3) the vagus nerve (n. X); and (4) the bulbar portion of the accessory nerve (n. XI). These will be considered collectively as the vagal system.

Course and Distribution of Nerves of the Vagal System

Nervus Intermedius

The nervus intermedius, the smaller of two divisions of the facial nerve, enters the internal acoustic meatus and proceeds laterally in the facial canal toward the medial wall of the middle ear cavity. The sensory ganglion (geniculate ganglion) is located at the angle of a sharp bend in the canal. From this point, some fibers of the nerve continue as the greater superficial petrosal nerve to the pterygopalatine ganglion. The rest of the nervus intermedius passes downward in the facial canal, but leaves it abruptly and crosses the tympanic cavity as the chorda tympani. Leaving the middle ear at the inner end of the petrotympanic fissure, the chorda tympani descends between the pterygoid muscles to join the lingual branch of the mandibular nerve. Some fibers of the chorda tympani are given off to the submandibular ganglion; the rest are distributed to taste receptors in the anterior two-thirds of the tongue.

Glossopharyngeal Nerve

The glossopharyngeal nerve leaves the skull through the jugular foramen at which point its two sensory ganglia, the superior and inferior petrosal, are located. The nerve passes downward and forward upon the surfaces of the stylopharyngeus and constrictor pharyngeus muscles to be distributed to the mucosa of the palatine tonsil, the fauces, and to the posterior one-third of the tongue.

BRANCHES OF THE GLOSSOPHARYNGEAL NERVE:

1. Tympanic (Jacobson's nerve): enters the tympanic plexus and

71

proceeds as the lesser superficial petrosal nerve to the otic ganglion.

2. Carotid: descends along the internal carotid artery to end in the carotid sinus and the carotid body.
3. Pharyngeal: enters the pharyngeal plexus with the vagus nerve and contributes motor fibers to the striated muscles of the pharynx.
4. Stylopharyngeal: to the stylopharyngeus muscle.
5. Lingual: sends taste and general sensory fibers to the posterior third of the tongue.

Vagus Nerve

The two sensory ganglia of the vagus nerve, the superior (jugular) and inferior (nodose), are located near the jugular foramen through which the nerve passes. The nerve courses vertically down the neck in the carotid sheath and enters the thorax, passing anterior to the subclavian artery on the right and anterior to the aortic arch on the left. Both nerves pass behind the roots of the lungs. The left nerve continues on the anterior side, the right on the posterior side of the esophagus, to reach the gastric plexus. Fibers diverge to the duodenum, liver, biliary ducts, spleen, kidneys, and to the small and large intestine as far as the splenic flexure.

BRANCHES OF THE VAGUS NERVE:

1. Auricular: to skin in the external auditory canal and a small sector of the pinna (the central connections of this branch may be to the trigeminal system).
2. Pharyngeal: to the pharyngeal plexus, along with the glossopharyngeal nerve. Is the chief motor nerve of pharynx and soft palate.
3. Superior laryngeal: internal branch is sensory to mucosa of larynx and epiglottis; external branch innervates inferior pharyngeal constrictor and cricothyroid muscles.
4. Recurrent laryngeal: on the left side the nerve loops around the aortic arch from before backwards; on the right it takes a similar course around the subclavian artery. Both nerves ascend in the laryngotracheal grooves and supply motor fibers to the intrinsic muscles of the larynx and sensory fibers to the mucosa below the vocal cords.

5. Cardiac (superior and inferior cervical cardiac rami and thoracic branches): enter the cardiac plexus on the wall of the heart with cardiac nerves from the sympathetic trunks.
6. Pericardial, bronchial, esophageal, and others branch through the celiac and superior mesenteric plexi to the abdominal viscera.

Bulbar Accessory Nerve

The bulbar accessory nerve is joined with the vagus nerve and forms a portion of the pharyngeal branches.

Motor Portion of the Vagal System

The vagal system contains special visceral motor preganglionic parasympathetic and sensory fibers but there is no separation of bundles into dorsal and ventral nerve roots as in the spinal nerves. All fibers enter and leave the medulla in a series of rootlets arranged in a longitudinal row posterior to the olive (Fig. 27).

The cells of the nucleus ambiguus are lower motor neurons. Their axons enter the glossopharyngeal and vagus nerves to furnish the motor innervation of the striated branchiomeric musculature of the soft palate, the pharynx, and the larynx (see Fig. 27).

Lower motor neuron lesions of the vagal system may cause difficulty in swallowing (dysphagia); regurgitation of fluids through the nose; difficulty in producing vocal sounds (dysphonia); and development of a nasal quality of consonant sounds (dysarthria). Unilateral paralysis of the vagus nerve produces flattening of the palatal arch on that side and, on phonation, the uvula is drawn to the nonparalyzed side. One of the recurrent nerves may be injured inadvertently during operations on the thyroid gland resulting in transient or permanent hoarseness. Paralysis of both recurrent nerves produces stridor and dyspnea which may necessitate tracheotomy.

Parasympathetic Portion of the Vagal System

The *dorsal motor nucleus of the vagus nerve* consists of nerve cell bodies whose axons leave the medulla and are distributed to ganglia located in the head, neck, thorax, and abdomen. The ganglia are located close to or within the viscera which they innervate and they send short fibers directly to the smooth muscle and gland cells of

73

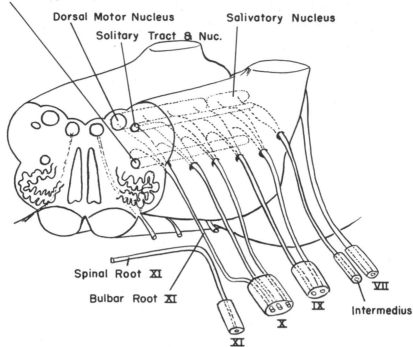

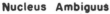

Nucleus Ambiguus

Dorsal Motor Nucleus   **Salivatory Nucleus**

Solitary Tract & Nuc.

Spinal Root XI

Bulbar Root XI

VII

IX

Intermedius

X

XI

FIGURE 27. Attachments of the nervus intermedius (VII), the glossopharyngeal (IX), vagus (X), and bulbar accessory (XI) nerves to the upper portion of the medulla. The internal course of their motor, parasympathetic and sensory fibers is indicated.

these organs. The fibers that arise in the dorsal motor nucleus are referred to as preganglionic fibers; those proceeding from the ganglia to muscle and gland cells are postganglionic.

At the rostral end of the dorsal motor nuclear column is a group of neurons called the *salivatory nucleus;* activity of its cells stimulates secretion by the salivary glands. The cells in the superior part of the salivatory nucleus send their preganglionic fibers to the nervus intermedius, while those in the inferior part of the nucleus send preganglionic fibers to the glossopharyngeal nerve. (see Fig. 27). Some of the preganglionic fibers entering the nervus intermedius terminate in the pterygopalatine ganglion. This parasympathetic ganglion sends postganglionic fibers to the lacrimal gland and to the mucosal glands of the palate, pharynx, and posterior nasal chambers. Other preganglionic fibers of the nervus intermedius end in the submandibular ganglion which sends postganglionic fibers to the submandibular and sublingual salivary glands. Preganglionic fibers of the glossopharyngeal nerve end in the otic ganglion, the parasympathetic ganglion which innervates the parotid gland.

74

The dorsal motor nucleus furnishes the preganglionic fibers of the vagus nerve, the largest and most important parasympathetic nerve of the body. Ganglion cells receiving terminals of the vagus nerve are found in the autonomic plexuses of the walls of the cervical, thoracic, and abdominal viscera. Stimulation of vagal parasympathetic fibers slows the heart rate; constricts the smooth muscle of the bronchial tree; stimulates the glands of the bronchial mucosa; promotes peristalsis in the gastrointestinal tract; relaxes the pyloric and ileocolic sphincters; and stimulates the secretion of gastric and pancreatic juices.

Sensory Portion of the Vagal System

The sensory fibers of the vagus and glossopharyngeal nerves have their cell bodies in the sensory ganglia which are attached to these nerves near the base of the skull. The geniculate ganglion, located at the external genu of the facial nerve, contains the cell bodies of the sensory fibers of the nervus intermedius. After entering the medulla in the dorsolateral sulcus, all sensory fibers of the vagal system pass directly into the solitary tract. The fibers turn in a caudal direction and give off terminal branches to the nucleus of the solitary tract as they descend (see Fig. 27).

The sense of taste, initiated by chemical stimulation of special receptor cells in the taste buds of the tongue, is carried to the rostral portion of the solitary tract by sensory fibers of the nervus intermedius and the glossopharyngeal nerves. The nervus intermedius, through its chorda tympani branch, receives the gustatory stimuli from the anterior two-thirds of the tongue; the glossopharyngeal, from the posterior one-third. A small number of taste buds located on the epiglottis receive innervation from the vagus nerve. Secondary fibers (the ascending gustatory tract) from the nucleus of the solitary tract are presumed to cross and ascend through the brain stem on the medial aspect of the medial lemniscus to the VPM nucleus of the thalamus. Thalamic fibers go to a cortical area for taste recognition located in the opercular part of the postcentral gyrus.

The glossopharyngeal and vagus nerves supply the afferent fibers of touch and pain senses to the mucosa of the posterior part of the soft palate, auditory tube, pharynx, larynx, and trachea. Touch fibers, whose nerve cell bodies are in the sensory ganglia of these nerves, enter the solitary tract along with the special sensory fibers of taste. Most of the touch fibers from this area are contained in the vagus nerve. Pain stimuli from the region of the pharynx are carried in the glossopharyngeal nerve, but after reaching the brain stem, these fibers descend in the spinal root of the trigeminal nerve instead of passing to the solitary tract.

The vagus nerve also conducts sensory stimuli from the heart, bronchi, esophagus, stomach, small intestine, and ascending colon. Vagal stimulation may be responsible for the indescribably, unpleasant sensation of nausea, but otherwise, afferent impulses from viscera are not recognized consciously when they are conducted by the vagal route. Visceral pain is transmitted by the anterolateral system of the spinal cord. The chief function of the nontaste, afferent fibers of the vagal system concerns the operation of visceral reflexes.

Reflexes of the Vagal System

Salivary-Taste Reflex

The secretory function of the vagal system is illustrated by the salivary-taste reflex. When a drop of weak acid is placed on the tongue, the salivary glands increase their output of saliva. The afferent stimulus is carried by the facial nerve to the nucleus of the solitary tract by taste fibers. Connecting fibers from this nucleus go to the superior and inferior salivatory nuclei of the facial and glossopharyngeal nerve stimulating parasympathetic neurons which supply the salivary glands.

Carotid Sinus Reflex

Increased blood pressure stimulates special baroreceptors in the wall of the carotid sinus and sends impulses over fibers of the glossopharyngeal nerve to the solitary tract. Connections from the solitary tract, or its nucleus, to the dorsal motor nucleus complete a reflex arc which slows the heart rate. Simultaneously, other reflex connections are made to a diffuse vasomotor center located in the reticular formation of the medulla. Inhibition of the vasomotor center, whose fibers descend to sympathetic neurons of the spinal cord, produces vasodilation of peripheral blood vessels and further reduces the blood pressure. Some individuals with hypersensitive carotid sinus reflexes are subject to attacks of syncope brought on by light external pressure over the sinus.

Carotid Body Reflex

The carotid body contains special chemoreceptors which respond to changes in the carbon dioxide and oxygen content of the circulating blood. Stimulation is carried to the solitary tract by the glossopharyngeal nerve. Fibers then go to the respiratory center of the medulla where they influence the rate of respiration. The respiratory center consists of diffusely arranged cells of the reticular formation with reticulospinal fibers descending to the lower motor neurons of the phrenic and intercostal nerves.

Propagation of nerve impulses over the reticulospinal fibers of the respiratory center produces inspiration. As the lungs become inflated, stretch receptors in the walls of bronchioles discharge impulses which ascend to the medulla through the vagus nerve. Connecting neurons reach the respiratory center and, by inhibition, temporarily arrest the inspiratory phase of respiration. The respiratory center is dependent on impulses descending from the pons for maintenance of the rhythm. The voluntary motor system can control respiration such as in singing or talking.

Cough Reflex

Coughing is usually a response to irritation of the larynx, trachea, or bronchial tree, but it may also be produced at times by irritation of vagus nerve fibers in other locations including the fibers that supply the external auditory canal or the tympanic membrane. Afferent impulses reach the solitary tract by way of the vagus nerve. Connections are made to the respiratory center to bring about forced expiration. At the same time, fibers going to the nucleus ambiguus cause efferent impulses to descend to the muscles of the larynx and pharynx.

Gag Reflex

Touching the posterior wall of the pharynx is followed by constriction and elevation of the pharynx. The afferent fibers for this reflex are sensory fibers of the glossopharyngeal nerve. After entering the solitary tract, synaptic connections are made with the nucleus ambiguus which sends efferent fibers to the striated muscles of the pharynx.

77

Vomiting Reflex

Forceful emptying of the stomach is brought about by relaxation of the gastroesophageal sphincter and contraction of the muscles of the anterior abdominal wall which expel gastric contents. At the same time, inspiration is arrested by closure of the glottis. The stimulus, which may arise in any part of the gut innervated by the vagus, is sent to the nucleus of the solitary tract by sensory fibers of the vagus nerve. From here, impulses go to the dorsal motor nucleus, to initiate the parasympathetic responses, and to the nucleus ambiguus to close the glottis. The diaphragm and the abdominal muscles are recruited by impulses which descend from the reticular formation of the medulla to reach the appropriate lower motor neurons in the spinal cord.

A general elevation of intracranial pressure often causes vomiting. This is attributed to increased pressure on the floor of the fourth ventricle, and it may also occur if there is localized pressure on the medulla.

12
Cranial Nerves of the Pons and Midbrain

ABDUCENS NERVE (NERVE VI)

The abducens nerve, arising from its nucleus beneath the fourth ventricle in the pons, supplies the motor fibers of the *lateral rectus muscle* of the eye. Leaving the brain stem anteriorally at the junction of the medulla and pons, the nerve passes along the floor of the posterior fossa of the skull to reach the lateral wall of the cavernous sinus. Prolonged elevation of intracranial pressure from any cause may damage the abducens nerve. Sustaining such damage makes it impossible to turn the eye outward. The unopposed pull of the medial rectus muscle causes the eye to turn inward (adduction) and produces *internal strabismus,* or squint. Since images do not fall on corresponding points of the left and right retinae, they cannot be properly fused. The result is *diplopia,* or double vision, which the patient seeks to minimize by turning the head to one side. Weakness of one external rectus muscle may only become apparent when the patient attempts to turn the eyes to one side and is unable to move the affected eye laterally from the middle position. With bilateral abducens nerve paralysis, neither eye can be moved in a lateral direction past the midposition.

TROCHLEAR NERVE (NERVE IV)

The nucleus of the trochlear nerve is located anterior to the central gray matter in the region of the inferior colliculus. The fibers of the nerve descend slightly and curve around the central gray matter. The fibers decussate in the anterior medullary velum and make their exit from the posterior surface of the tectum caudal to the inferior colliculus. The trochlear nerve innervates the superior oblique muscle. Isolated lesions of the trochlear nerve are uncommon and the symptoms are inconspicuous. The ability to turn the eye outward and downward is impaired.

OCULOMOTOR NERVE (NERVE III)

The nucleus of the oculomotor nerve is located anterior to the central gray matter in the region of the superior colliculus. The fibers course anteriorally, some penetrating the lateral portion of the red nucleus and the medial portion of the cerebral peduncle. After its exit from the brain stem at the interpeduncular fossa, the nerve passes close to the arteries of the circulus arteriosus (circle of Willis) which is an anastomotic circuit at the base of the brain. An aneurysm (saccular dilation) in one of the arteries in this region may compress the oculomotor nerve. Tumor or hemorrhage may force the inferior margin of the temporal lobe of the cerebrum under the edge of the tentorium cerebelli and exert pressure on the oculomotor nerve as it crosses the tentorium beside the dorsum sellae of the sphenoid bone.

The oculomotor nerve innervates the *medial, superior* and *inferior recti,* the *inferior oblique,* and the *levator palpebrae superioris.* It also supplies the *preganglionic parasympathetic fibers to the ciliary ganglion* whose postganglionic fibers innervate the *ciliary muscle for accommodation* and the *sphincter muscle of the iris* which constricts the pupil.

Complete paralysis of the oculomotor nerve results in: (1) outward deviation (abduction) of the eye (*external strabismus*) and inability to turn the eye inward; (2) *ptosis,* or drooping of the upper eyelid, with inability to raise the lid voluntarily; and (3) dilation of the pupil (*mydriasis*) because of the unopposed action of the radial muscle fibers of the iris which are supplied by the sympathetic system. Incomplete lesions produce partial effects. There may be some weakness of all functions, or one symptom may appear without the others, for example, dilation of the pupil without paralysis of eye movements.

The upper motor neurons which descend as the corticoreticulo-oculomotor pathways to motor nuclei of nerves III, IV, and VI cross in the pons and make connections with all three nuclei to bring about cooperative, or conjugate, movements of both eyes. Upper motor neuronal lesions, therefore, usually do not affect one nerve without involving the others. The cortex of the left frontal lobe controls voluntary deviation of the eyes to the right. Destructive lesions above the crossing of the corticomesencephalic tract cause loss of the ability to turn the eyes voluntarily to the side opposite the lesion. Following such a lesion, the predominating influence of the unaffected corticoreticulo-oculomotor tracts may cause both eyes to be deviated to the side of the lesion so that the patient "looks at his lesion."

FACIAL NERVE (NERVE VII)

The motor division of the seventh cranial nerve is considered to be the facial nerve proper, its sensory and parasympathetic components (nervus intermedius) having been included with the vagal system. The facial is the motor nerve of the muscles of facial expression (*mimetic muscles*). Through the action of the orbicularis oculi muscle, the facial nerve closes the eyelid and protects the eye.

The facial nerve proceeds from the pontocerebellar angle, enters the facial canal, leaves the skull by the stylomastoid foramen, and courses through the substance of the parotid gland behind the ramus of the mandible where it divides into branches which fan out to all parts of the face and scalp.

An interruption of the facial nerve causes total paralysis of the muscles of facial expression on that side. The muscles of one side of the face sag and the normal lines around the lips, nose, and forehead are "ironed out." On attempting to smile, the corner of the mouth is drawn to the opposite side. Saliva may drip from the corner of the mouth. The cheek may puff out in expiration because the buccinator muscle is paralyzed. The patient's inability to close his eyes leads to irritation and predisposes to infection, so it is advisable for him to wear an eye mask or to have the lids closed by sutures. It is not uncommon for the facial nerve to become paralyzed overnight without any known cause, a condition known as Bell's palsy. Fortunately, most of these patients recover spontaneously in one or two months.

There are no stretch reflexes available for testing the superficial musculature of the face so these cannot serve as a point of distinction in upper motor neurons involving facial fibers of the corticobulbar tract. A supranuclear lesion of this type can usually be recognized by other means. Nearly all of the upper motor neurons going to those cells of the facial nucleus which supply the lower part of the face below the angle of the eye are crossed fibers; uncrossed as well as crossed fibers are sent to motor cells for the upper part of the face

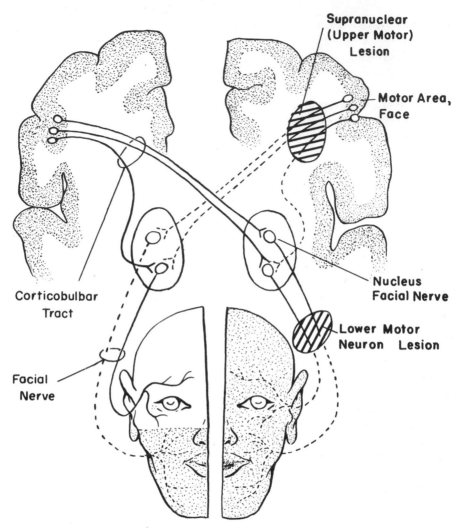

FIGURE 28. The shaded areas of the face show the distribution of facial muscles paralyzed after a supranuclear lesion of the corticobulbar tract, and after a lower motor neuron lesion of the facial nerve.

(Fig. 28). An upper motor neuron lesion, therefore, interrupts all of the voluntary control fibers for lower facial muscles, but leaves an uncrossed connection **open** for willed movements of the upper facial muscles. As a result the upper part of the face is spared from paralysis.

When paralysis is due to injury to upper motor neurons rather than to the facial nerve itself or its nucleus, involuntary contraction of the muscles of facial expression is still possible. By utilizing extrapyramidal circuits, a spontaneous grin may occur by utilizing muscles which cannot be moved voluntarily.

TRIGEMINAL NERVE (NERVE V)

The trigeminal nerve is a mixed nerve with a large motor root supplying the *muscles of mastication* and an even larger sensory root distributed to the mouth, nasal cavity, orbit, and anterior one-half of the scalp.

Motor Division of Nerve V

Fibers from the masticator, or motor nucleus, in the lateral tegmentum of the pons enter the mandibular branch of the fifth nerve and innervate the temporalis, masseter, and medial and lateral pterygoid muscles (other less important muscles are also supplied). Peripheral lesions of this portion of the nerve cause atrophy and weakness which can be recognized by feeling the size and tautness of the masseter muscles as the jaws are clenched. Fasciculations may also be seen in the denervated muscle fibers. Owing to the action of the pterygoid muscles which draw the mandible forward and toward the midline, there is deviation of the chin in the direction of the paralyzed side when the jaws are opened. Each motor nucleus receives upper motor neurons from both the left and the right motor areas of the cortex, and supranuclear lesions confined to one side do not produce any marked effects. The jaw jerk is a stretch reflex obtained by tapping the middle of the chin while the mouth is slightly open. The normal response, which is usually a minimal one becomes exaggerated after upper motor neuron lesions.

Sensory Division of Nerve V

The trigeminal (semilunar, gasserian) ganglion contains the cell bodies of the afferent fibers of the fifth nerve with the unique exception of the proprioceptive fibers from neuromuscular spindles, whose cell bodies are in the mesencephalic nucleus of the nerve. Pain and temperature fibers turn caudally after entering the pons and form the spinal root of the trigeminal nerve, giving off terminal branches to the nucleus of the spinal tract of V as they descend through the pons and medulla. Fibers arising from cells of the nucleus of the spinal tract cross to the opposite side of the brain stem in a

83

diffuse pattern as the *anterior trigeminothalamic tract* and ascend to the medial part of the ventral posteromedial (VPM) nucleus of the thalamus from which thalamocortical fibers are projected to the postcentral gyrus. Similar crossing fibers (the *posterior trigeminothalamic tract*) are given off from the principal sensory nucleus (Fig. 29). The name trigeminal lemniscus is sometimes applied to all of the trigeminothalamic fibers, although they are never gathered into a distinct and separate bundle. In the medulla, the crossed pain and temperature fibers of the face are located near the medial lemniscus; as they reach the pons, they gradually shift laterally to join the lateral spinothalamic tract.

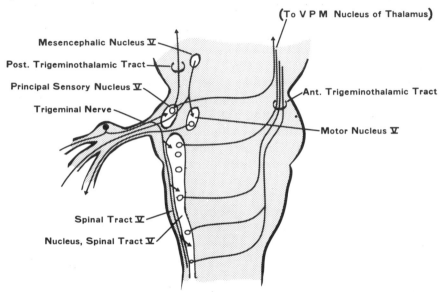

FIGURE 29. Connections of the sensory and motor fibers of the trigeminal nerve within the brain stem from posterior aspect. The nuclei are shown on one side for the sake of clarity.

Lesions in the lateral part of the medulla or lower pons which damage the spinal tract of the trigeminal nerve are likely to include the lateral spinothalamic tract also. This causes *alternating analgesia*: loss of pain and temperature sense on the same side of the face as the lesion, and loss of pain and temperature sense on the opposite side of the body beginning at the neck. In the upper pons and midbrain, the fibers of the pain-temperature and touch systems are all close together, and in these regions one lesion produces anesthesia of the opposite side of the body including the face.

When the cornea is touched by a foreign body, the *corneal reflex* produces prompt closing of the eyelids. Sensory fibers entering the upper part of the spinal tract of the trigeminal nerve synapse with cells of the nucleus of the spinal tract which send axons to the nucleus of the facial nerve (see Fig. 29). Motor fibers of the facial nerve then activate the orbicularis oculi muscle to close the eye. Connecting fibers go to both facial nuclei to close both eyes. The response on the side which is stimulated is the direct corneal reflex; that in the other eye is the consensual corneal reflex. Interrupting the trigeminal nerve abolishes both responses. A consensual but no direct reflex will be obtained if the ipsilateral facial nerve is destroyed; but at the same time, reflex connections are made with autonomic neurons to produce increased lacrimation.

Tic douloureux, or *trigeminal neuralgia,* is a disorder characterized by attacks of unbearably severe pain over the distribution of one or more branches of the trigeminal nerve. A small trigger zone may be present; stimulation of it sets off a painful paroxysm. No cause for the disease has been discovered.

13
Hearing

THE AUDITORY SYSTEM

The eighth cranial nerve is the original sensory nerve of the semicircular canals of fish—an effective mechanism for maintaining equilibrium and orientation in space.

The auditory organ, initially the lagena and then the cochlea, have been developed in the labyrinth of the land vertebrates. Because of this evolutionary change, a new exteroceptive division of the eighth nerve appeared to serve the auditory function. Thus, the eighth nerve has two components—a vestibular and a cochlear division. Both are so distinct in their function and anatomical relationship that they could almost be considered as separate cranial nerves.

The auditory apparatus consists of three components—the external, the middle, and the internal ear. The *tympanic membrane* of the external ear receives the airborne vibrations. The chain of three ossicles (*malleus, incus,* and *stapes*) in the middle ear is an amplifier as well as an impedance-matching device which decreases the amount of energy loss in going from the air to the perilymph behind the oval window. The internal ear, or *cochlea,* is a tube resembling a snail shell, about 3.5 cm long, and exhibiting 2½ turns. The central pillar or *modiolus* provides the bony support for the *bony spiral lamina* which partially divides the cochlea into two fluid filled (perilymph) chambers—the *scala vestibuli* and the *scala tympani.* The basilar membrane completes the separation of the scalae. A subdivision of the scala vestibuli, the scala media (cochlear duct), is bordered by the vestibular membrane on the upper surface. The cochlear duct contains *endolymph* and is bordered by the *organ of Corti* which contains the sensory epithelium or the hair cells. The piston action of the stapes produces an instantaneous pressure wave in the perilymph of the *scala vestibuli* which travels to the *helicotrema* (the apical connection between the scala vestibuli and tympani) in 25 microseconds. A traveling wave is set up on the basilar membrane, as a result of shearing forces produced by the pressure wave in the perilymph of the scala vestibuli. The mechanical properties of the basilar membrane (upon which the organ of Corti is located) change gradually, progressing from base to apex while permitting a spatial resolution of frequencies by the hair cells in the organ of Corti. The basilar membrane increases in width from the base of the cochlea to the apex. The pressure waves after traversing through the scala media, across the basilar membrane, and through the scala tympani, are dampened at the *round window*. The pressure waves cause a vibration of the basilar membrane which stimulates the hair cells of the organ of Corti. The hair cells serve as mechanoreceptors in which the mechanical energy (pressure waves) is transduced into a stimulation potential which is received by the closely applied dendritic processes of the spiral ganglion cells. The *spiral ganglion*, located in the modiolus of the cochlea, contains the bipolar cells of the cochlear division of the eighth nerve.

The organ of Corti serves as an audio-frequency analyzer. It is tonotopically organized so that the highest tones (highest in pitch and frequency) maximally stimulate the hair cells in the most basal portion of the cochlea. The tones of lowest pitch maximally stimulate the most apical hair cells. Tones or sounds in between stimulate the hair cells in the intermediate portion of the basilar membrane.

The Auditory Pathway

The cochlear nerve enters the brain stem at the junction of the medulla and pons. As it attaches to the brain stem, the nerve clings to the lateral side of the inferior cerebellar peduncle and enters the *posterior (dorsal) and anterior (ventral) cochlear nuclei.* The entering nerve fibers bifurcate and make synapses with both cochlear nuclei. The nuclei are tonotopically organized. Three projections, the acoustic striae, arise from the cochlear nuclei to relay the information centrally and rostrally. The *dorsal acoustic stria* originates from the posterior cochlear nucleus, passes over the inferior cerebellar peduncle, and crosses to join the contralateral *lateral lemniscus* (Fig. 30). The two other projections arise from the anterior cochlear nucleus. The *intermediate acoustic stria* takes a course which is similar to

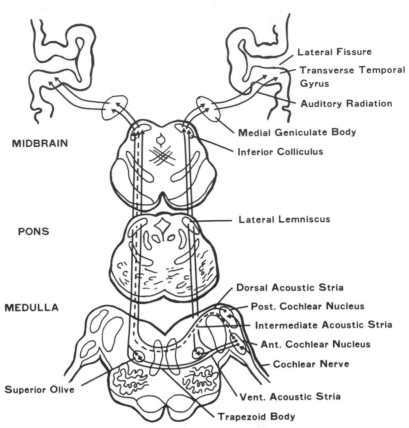

FIGURE 30. The auditory pathways.

that of the dorsal stria. The *ventral acoustic stria* takes a different route and passes anterior to the inferior cerebellar peduncle to terminate in the ipsilateral and contralateral *superior olivary nuclei* and the *nuclei of the trapezoid body.* These nuclear groups are tonotopically organized. They project fibers into the ipsilateral and contralateral lateral lemnisci. Fibers in the lateral lemniscus ascend through the brain stem to terminate primarily in the *nucleus of the inferior colliculus* (tonotopically organized). Some of the fibers terminate in small nuclear groups, the nuclei of the lateral lemniscus, which are intermingled with the lateral lemniscus. A few fibers of the lateral lemniscus pass directly to the medial geniculate body as the central acoustic tract; most of them terminate in the *nucleus of the inferior colliculus* which sends axons to the *medial geniculate* body through the *brachium of the inferior colliculus.*

The medial geniculate bodies are the final sensory relay stations of the hearing path, a special sensory nucleus of the thalamus. The

88

efferent connection of the medial geniculate body to the temporal lobe forms the auditory radiation which goes to the *anterior transverse temporal gyrus (gyrus of Heschl)* located on the dorsal surface of the superior temporal convolution and partly buried in the lateral fissure. This relatively small cortical area, area 41, is the primary auditory receptive area. When auditory impulses arrive at area 41, a noise is "heard," but the intelligent recognition of a particular sound depends on the auditory associative cortex. Whether or not the medial geniculate body and superior temporal gyrus are tonotopically organized has not been resolved.

Descending efferent fibers have been found recently in all parts of the auditory pathway. It is believed that they function as feedback loops. The olivocochlear bundle (from the superior olive to the ipsilateral and contralateral organ of Corti by the vestibular nerve) may have an inhibitory action on the impulses from the cochlea.

Bilateral Representation of the Ears
in Each Temporal Lobe

Above the level at which the cochlear nerve enters the brain stem, the hearing pathway is made up of crossed and uncrossed fibers, the majority of which are crossed. Opportunity for auditory information to be redistributed in both crossed and uncrossed fashion exists at many levels of the brain stem. Fibers crossing from one side to the other occur between the superior olivary nuclei, the nuclei of the trapezoid body, the nuclei of the lateral lemnisci, and the nuclei of the inferior colliculi. Each lateral lemniscus, therefore, conducts stimuli from both ears. A lesion of the right lateral lemniscus, or of the right anterior transverse temporal gyrus, stops some impulses from both ears, but does not interfere with other impulses from both ears going to the cortex of the left hemisphere. No appreciable hearing deficit, other than inability to localize directions of sounds, is produced. Deafness in one ear usually signifies trouble in the acoustic nerve, the cochlea, or the sound-conducting apparatus of that side. The eighth nerve can be damaged bilaterally by toxic effects of some drugs, the most notorious being streptomycin, quinine, and aspirin.

Hearing Defects from Nerve Damage and from
Mechanical Obstruction

Hearing loss and tinnitus (ringing or roaring in the ear) are common symptoms of eighth nerve disorder, but they also may be caused by middle ear disease, or by wax in the external meatus. Tuning fork examinations are helpful in distinguishing deafness caused by damage to the nerve or cochlea from conduction deafness which refers to the interference with the transmission of sound waves to the cochlea. The Rinne test compares the patient's ability to hear a vibrating fork by bone conduction and by air conduction. The base of the fork is placed over the mastoid process of the skull. When it can no longer be heard, it is removed and the tines are held in front of the ear. A normal person continues to hear by air conduction after bone conduction ceases. In nerve deafness, both are diminished but air conduction remains better than bone conduction. In conduction deafness, bone conduction is better than air conduction. The Weber test is performed by placing the base of the fork on the midline of the skull and asking the patient which ear hears the louder sound. In conduction deafness, the sound is heard better in the defective ear; in nerve deafness it seems louder in the normal ear. Electronic audiometers have an important role in testing hearing since pure tones may be used at controlled intensities. Receivers for both air and bone conduction are available. It is possible to graph the results of these tests on the right and left ear for both air and bone conduction. Conduction deafness is indicated by a reception impairment in the lower frequencies of pure tones in the air conduction test. In nerve deafness tested in the same manner, the threshold deficit occurs in the reception of tones in the higher frequencies.

Auditory Reflexes

Auditory reflexes are operated by side branches from the main auditory pathway. Many of these synapse in the reticular formation to evoke autonomic responses. The *superior olive* sends a bundle of fibers to the vicinity of the nucleus of the abducens nerve which continues, through the medial longitudinal fasciculus, to the nuclei of the oculomotor and trochlear nerves. These connections bring about conjugate movements of the eyes in response to a sound. Other fibers from the *tectum* continue into the spinal cord as components of the *tectospinal tract*. These fibers terminate on lower motor neurons in the cervical spinal cord supplying the muscles of the head and neck which respond to sound.

14

The Vestibular System

The vestibular part of the eighth nerve has its peripheral endings on the *hair cells of both the maculae of the utricle and saccule,* and on the *cristae in the ampullae of the three semicircular canals.* The nerve furnishes proprioceptive afferent fibers for coordinated reflexes of the eyes, neck, and body for maintaining equilibrium in accordance with the posture and movement of the head.

The Vestibular Nerve and Its Central Connections

Axons of bipolar cells of the vestibular ganglion pass through the internal auditory canal and reach the upper medulla in company with the cochlear nerve. Most of the fibers of the vestibular nerve bifurcate into ascending and descending branches and terminate in the vestibular nuclei which are clustered in the lateral part of the floor of the fourth ventricle (Fig. 31): the *medial vestibular nucleus* (of Schwalbe), *lateral vestibular nucleus* (of Deiter), *superior vestibular nucleus* (of Bechterew), and *inferior vestibular nucleus* (descending, spinal).

The afferent fibers innervating the cristae of the semicircular canals terminate in the medial and superior vestibular nuclei primarily, while those from the maculae terminate in the lateral and inferior nuclei. The *canals* respond to *angular movements of acceleration and deceleration,* while the *utriculus* is concerned with *gravitational motion* (linear acceleration) concerning the *position of the head in*

91

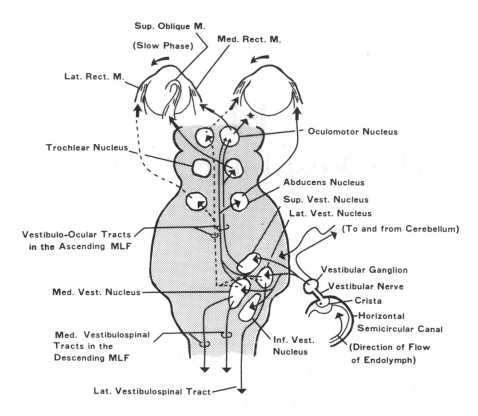

Sup. Oblique M.

(Slow Phase)

Med. Rect. M.

Lat. Rect. M.

Trochlear Nucleus

Oculomotor Nucleus

Abducens Nucleus

Sup. Vest. Nucleus

Lat. Vest. Nucleus

(To and from Cerebellum)

Vestibulo-Ocular Tracts in the Ascending MLF

Vestibular Ganglion

Vestibular Nerve

Crista

Horizontal Semicircular Canal

Med. Vest. Nucleus

Med. Vestibulospinal Tracts in the Descending MLF

Inf. Vest. Nucleus

(Direction of Flow of Endolymph)

Lat. Vestibulospinal Tract

FIGURE 31. Vestibular pathways. Nystagmus induced by centripetal flow of endolymph in a horizontal semicircular canal is indicated. The dotted lines show the probable route of activating stimuli. MLF = medial longitudinal fasciculus.

space. The *saccule* may be a sensor for *vibratory stimuli* and may also influence *eye movements.*

A few primary fibers of the vestibular nerve pass directly to the cerebellum, ending in the cortex of the flocculonodular lobe. Connections are made within the cerebellum to the *nucleus fastigii* which gives rise to the *fastigiobulbar tract* (tract of Russell). The fibers of this tract are crossed and uncrossed and terminate in the vestibular nuclei (primarily the lateral vestibular nucleus) and on the hair cells of the labyrinth. As they pass from the cerebellum, they loop around the superior cerebellar peduncle to form the *uncinate fasciculus* (hook bundle). Other fibers from the fastigial nucleus which are uncrossed pass to and from the cerebellum on the medial side of the inferior cerebellar peduncle and constitute a portion of the peduncle sometimes referred to as the *juxtarestiform body.* An additional efferent component arises in the lateral vestibular nucleus primarily, which terminates on the vestibular hair cells. It is believed that the *vestibular efferent fibers* exhibit a central influence on the receptors of the membranous labyrinth.

The Vestibulospinal Tracts

Two vestibulospinal tracts arise from the vestibular nuclei. The lateral tract (uncrossed) comes from the lateral vestibular nucleus; the medial tract, (which is primarily uncrossed) comes chiefly from the medial vestibular nucleus. The lateral vestibulospinal tract extends to the sacral level of the cord. The medial vestibulospinal tract extends through the cervical level. Both tracts terminate almost exclusively upon interneurons in laminae VII and VIII which in turn synapse upon the alpha and gamma lower motor neurons (see Chapter 4). Impulses descending in these tracts assist the local myotactic reflexes and reinforce the tonus of the extensor muscles of the trunk and limbs, producing enough extra force to support the body against gravity and maintain an upright posture.

An animal whose brain stem has been transected at the midbrain displays decerebrate rigidity with the legs held stiffly in extension. To produce *decerebrate rigidity*, there must be normal gravitational pull on the maculae of the utricles and the vestibular nuclei, vestibulospinal tracts, and dorsal roots must be intact. It is probable that decerebration abolishes the effect of certain descending fiber tracts and allows tonic labyrinthine reflexes to send a continuous discharge to the spinal cord over the vestibulospinal tracts. Decerebrate rigidity in its fully developed form is rarely seen in humans. Changes in tonus somewhat similar to decerebrate rigidity may appear in the muscles of the legs after transverse injury to the thoracic portion of the spinal cord. Complete transverse lesions usually result in paraplegia in flexion with the legs held in a permanently flexed position. Paraplegia in extension, with rigidity of the extensor muscles of the legs, occurs after incomplete lesions which spare the anterior funiculi. However, it is not certain whether the increase in extensor tonus is due to vestibulospinal or to reticulospinal fibers which are also located in the ventral part of the spinal cord.

The Vestibulo-ocular Pathways

The vestibular system is extremely important in controlling *conjugate eye movements* reflexly in response to head movement and to the position of the head in space. Fibers from the superior, medial, and to a lesser extent, the lateral and inferior vestibular nuclei project rostrally in the *medial longitudinal fasciculus.* The projections from the superior nucleus are uncrossed, while those from the other vestibular nuclei are both crossed and uncrossed. The fibers synapse on the somatic motor nuclei of the cranial nerves *(abducens, trochlear, and oculomotor)* that supply the extraocular muscles. Fibers from the MLF, (that perhaps indirectly influence eye movements) also project to several small nuclear groups located in the vicinity of the oculomotor nuclear complex and the pretectal area. These include the interstitial nucleus of Cajal, nucleus of Darkschewitsch, nucleus of the posterior commissure, and possibly thalamic nuclei. Vestibular reflexes, in cooperation with certain reflexes of the optic system, enable the eyes to remain fixed on stationary objects while the head and body are moving. Turning the head slightly to the right causes a small flow of endolymph in the horizontal semicircular canals. The flow is directed to the left because the fluid's inertia makes it lag behind the movement of the head. Vestibular impulses are sent to the abducens and oculomotor nuclei and the eyes are turned to the left the proper distance to keep the fields of vision unchanged.

In order to produce reflexly *left horizontal conjugate deviation* of the eyes, stimuli travel through the MLF to excite the left abducens nucleus (to innervate the left lateral rectus muscle) and to the right oculomotor nucleus (to innervate the right medial rectus muscle) (see Fig. 31). Simultaneously, the MLF must inhibit the innervation to the left medial rectus and the right lateral rectus muscles.

Vestibular Nystagmus

If stimulation of hair cells in the appropriate ampulla of the semicircular canal is persistent, the eyes draw slowly to the left until they reach a limit and then jerk quickly to the right. These movements are repeated in rapid succession producing tremor-like oscillations of the eyes known as nystagmus. The *direction of nystagmus* is designated according to the direction of the *fast component,* although this is opposite to the movement induced by stimulation from the semicircular canal. The mechanism responsible for the component of nystagmus is not understood, but it probably is self-contained within the vestibular nuclei.

A *rotation test* for nystagmus may be performed by whirling the subject in a revolving chair, the head being tilted forward 30 degrees to bring the horizontal canals parallel with the floor. Movement is stopped abruptly after 10 or 12 turns. Momentum causes the endolymph to continue to flow in the direction in which the head had been turning even though the head is now stationary. The induced nystagmus lasts about 30 seconds in normal individuals. If rotation has been to the left, endolymph flows to the left and the slow component of the nystagmus is to the left. Since the quick component is to the right, it is properly called "nystagmus to the right." With a special chair designed to rotate the subject in any plane, it is possible to test each of the three semicircular canals individually.

Caloric, or *thermal*, *tests* of nystagmus permit the vestibular system of each side to be tested separately. The subject is usually seated with the head tilted backwards about 60 degrees to bring the horizontal semicircular canal into a vertical plane, then the external auditory canal is douched with cold or hot water. Hot water warms the endolymph in the semicircular canal and causes it to rise. Stimulation of hair cells by the current flowing past the ampulla produces nystagmus. With hot water in the right ear the current goes to the left and the hystagmus has its slow component to the left, and quick to the right. If cold water is used, the current is reversed and nystagmus is in the opposite direction.

Irritation or destruction of the vestibule, vestibular nerve, or the vestibular nuclei commonly produces nystagmus and may also cause deviation of the eyes to one side. If the right vestibular nerve is severed, the influence of the remaining left vestibular apparatus is unbalanced and causes conjugate deviation of the eyes to the right. In a few weeks, this effect is overcome by the compensating influence of voluntary and visual reflex circuits. The quick component of nystagmus produced by an irritative lesion is usually toward the side of the lesion, but at times it may be difficult to distinguish effects of irritation on one side from those of destruction on the other. Although *horizontal nystagmus is the most common type*, vertical or rotatory forms of nystagmus also occur. Nystagmus is not due to a disturbance of the vestibular system in every instance; some types are produced by injuries to the cerebral cortex, optic reflex pathways, the cerebellum, or by toxic substances.

Sensory Aspects of Vestibular Stimulation

Fiber connections from the vestibular nuclei to the thalamus and cerebral cortex have been postulated but not demonstrated. However, stimulation of the vestibular apparatus, whether by motion of the body or by artificial means, produces definite conscious effects which take the form of a false sense of motion. Vertigo is a sensation of whirling. The individual himself may have a subjective feeling of rotation, or it may seem to him that external objects are spinning around. Feelings of giddiness, faintness, and lightheadedness may be vaguely described in somewhat similar terms, but they should not be mistaken for true vertigo. Ménière's syndrome is a disease of uncertain nature which is characterized by periodic attacks of severe vertigo, often accompanied by nausea and prostration. Tinnitus and impairment of hearing are included in the syndrome. Motion sickness during travel by air or sea is a familiar manifestation of prolonged and unusual stimulation of the vestibular apparatus.

15

The Cerebellum

The cerebellum is situated in the posterior cranial fossa. It is attached to the pons, medulla, and midbrain by the cerebellar peduncles which lie at the sides of the fourth ventricle on the ventral aspect of the cerebellum. The tentorium cerebelli, a transverse fold of the dura mater, stretches horizontally over the superior surface of the cerebellum and separates it from the overlying occipital lobes of the cerebrum. The surface of the cerebellum is corrugated by numerous parallel folds known as folia. A layer of gray matter, the cerebellar cortex, covers the surface and encloses an internal core of white matter. Four pair of *deep cerebellar nuclei* are buried within the cerebellum (see Fig. 22 and description in Chapter 5). From medial to lateral these consist of the *fastigial nucleus*, the *globose nucleus*, the *emboliform nucleus*, and the *dentate nucleus*.

PRIMARY SUBDIVISIONS OF THE CEREBELLUM

For descriptive purposes, the cerebellum is divided into two large lateral masses, the *cerebellar hemispheres,* which fuse near the midline with a narrow middle portion called the *vermis* because of its fancied resemblance to a worm. Detailed descriptions of the anatomical subdivisions of the hemispheres and vermis are complicated and inconsistent. To avoid confusion, it will be sufficient here to partition the entire cerebellum into three lobes:

1. The *flocculonodular lobe* (archicerebellum) consists of the paired flocculi, which are small appendages in the posterior

97

inferior region and the nodulus, which is the inferior part of the vermis.

2. The *anterior lobe* (paleocerebellum), of modest size, is the portion of the cerebellum which lies anterior to the primary sulcus.
3. The *posterior lobe* (neocerebellum) is the larger, or main part, of the cerebellum and is located between the other two lobes. It contains the major portions of the cerebellar hemispheres.

The flocculonodular lobe represents the cerebellar portion of the vestibular system and, phylogenically, is the oldest part of the cerebellum. The anterior lobe, particularly its vermis portion, receives most of the proprioceptive impulses of the spinocerebellar pathways and is also an early developed area of the cerebellum. The flocculonodular and the anterior lobes are the predominant regions in the primitive vertebrates. The posterior lobe receives the cerebellar connections of the cerebrum and has become greatly expanded in the mammals which have developed an extensive cerebral cortex.

The foregoing description presents the *transverse arrangement* of the cerebellum. This is based upon the formation of 10 rostrocaudally arranged lobules during embryological development and the formation of various transverse fissures. Currently, a more popular method of describing the cerebellum is based upon *longitudinal zonal patterns (sagittal)*. Simply put, this classification subdivides each half of the cerebellum into three mediolaterally arranged longitudinal strips: (1) *vermal region*, (2) *paravermal region*, and (3) *lateral (hemisphere) region*.

The Cerebellar Cortex

The cerebellar cortex consists of three layers (Fig. 32):

1. *Molecular layer* (outermost layer) which contains: two types of neurons, the *stellate and basket cells*, dendrites of Purkinje and Golgi type II cells, and axons (T-shaped parallel fibers) of the granule cells.
2. *Purkinje cell layer* (middle layer): these are very large flask-like neurons that have enormous dendritic arborizations (which extend up into the molecular layer) and long axons that synapse either upon deep cerebellar nuclei or vestibular nuclei.
3. *Granular layer* (innermost layer) which contains: numerous *granule cells* (neurons), *Golgi type II cells* (neurons), and *glomeruli* (complex synaptic nodules which contain axons of incoming mossy fibers, axons and dendrites of Golgi type II

98

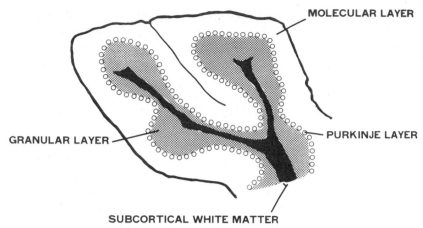

FIGURE 32. Cerebellar cortex.

cells, and dendrites of granule cells). Each glomerulus is en-wrapped by glial cells.

The intricate relationships between the various neurons of the cerebellar cortex are extremely complex and a discussion of this goes beyond the scope of this book. However, a few important features are essential to the understanding of how the cerebellum functions.

Afferents to the cerebellum terminate either in the granule cell layer (in the glomeruli) as *mossy fibers* or upon the dendrites of Purkinje cells as *climbing fibers*. Both inputs are excitatory. Excited granule cells can excite Purkinje cells, basket cells, stellate cells, and Golgi type II cells. In turn, the basket and stellate cells inhibit Purkinje and Golgi type II cells. The Golgi type II cells inhibit granule cells. Finally, *the Purkinje cells (the bottleneck for all information exiting from the cerebellar cortex) are inhibitory to the deep cerebellar nuclei. Consequently, of all the neurons whose cells reside within the cerebellar cortex, the granule cell is the only excitatory one.*

The Peduncles of the Cerebellum

The three, paired cerebellar peduncles are composed of large numbers of fibers entering and leaving the cerebellum to connect it with other parts of the nervous system.

The *inferior cerebellar peduncle* (restiform body) contains a single efferent tract, the fastigiobulbar, which goes to the vestibular nuclei and completes a vestibular circuit through the cerebellum. Afferent fibers are much more numerous. They reach the inferior cerebellar peduncle from four sources: (1) fibers from the vestibular nerve; (2) olivocerebellar fibers from the inferior olivary nuclei; (3) the posterior and rostral spinocerebellar tracts from the spinal cord; (4) dorsal arcuate fibers (cuneocerebellar tract) from the accessory cuneate nucleus which lies lateral to the nucleus cuneatus in the medulla. The dorsal arcuate fibers furnish the cerebellar connections or proprioceptive fibers (areas C1 to T5) which have ascended in the posterior funiculi of the cord; and (5) reticulocerebellar fibers.

The *middle cerebellar peduncle* (brachium pontis) consists almost entirely of crossed fibers from the pontine nuclei in the gray substance in the basal part of the pons (pontocerebellar or transverse pontine fibers).

The *superior cerebellar peduncle* (brachium conjunctivum) is the main efferent connection of the cerebellum. The dentatorubrothalamic system arises from the dentate and other roof nuclei and is distributed chiefly to the red nucleus, thalamus, and reticular formation. The fastigiobulbar tract also runs with the peduncle for a short distance before it enters the inferior cerebellar peduncle. As it leaves the cerebellum, the peduncle is joined by the only afferent tract—the anterior spinocerebellar tract.

THE SYNERGISTIC FUNCTION OF THE CEREBELLUM

The cerebellum is responsible for muscle synergy throughout the body. It coordinates the action of muscle groups and times their contractions so that movements are performed smoothly and accurately. Voluntary movements can proceed without assistance from the cerebellum, but such movements are clumsy and disorganized. Lack of motor skill as a result of cerebellar dysfunction is called *asynergia or cerebellar ataxia.*

Although the cerebellum receives large numbers of afferent fibers, conscious perception does not occur in the cerebellum, nor do its efferent fibers give rise to conscious sensations elsewhere in the brain.

Afferent and Efferent Pathways of the Cerebellum

The cortex of the cerebellum is furnished with an immediate account of the progress of motor activity by signals from many sources. First, it is informed of the commands being issued from the cerebral cortex and the pyramidal system by a simultaneous outflow of nerve impulses by three cerebrocerebellar systems. The most important of these is the corticopontocerebellar pathway. This is a crossed path connecting one cerebral hemisphere with the cerebellar hemisphere on the opposite side by way of the *corticopontine tract* and the *middle cerebellar peduncle* (Fig. 33). The other pathways

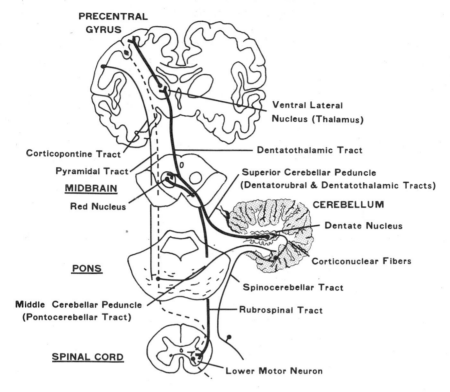

FIGURE 33. Cerebellar circuits. The spinocerebellar and corticopontocerebellar pathways to the cerebellum are represented by thin fibers. Thicker fibers show efferent paths from the dentate nucleus to the midbrain and thalamus. The pyramidal tract is shown as a dotted line.

originate primarily from motor areas of the cerebrum and include the *cerebro-olivocerebellar* and *cerebroreticulocerebellar systems.* Further communication received by the cerebellar cortex consists of instantaneous reports back from the muscles through the spinocerebellar tracts. All sensory modalities, including tactile, auditory, and visual stimuli, feed impulses to the cerebellum. These messages enter a vast pool of cortical neurons where, by unknown mechanisms, rapid correlations, and integrations must take place. In general, the vermis receives afferent input from the spinal cord, the flocculonodular lobe receives information from the vestibular system, and the cerebellar hemispheres receive input from the cerebral cortex.

101

After an evaluation of the afferent signals, the cerebellum is able to make an appropriate correction for any mistakes or inaccuracies of muscle activity. Nerve impulses are dispatched from the dentate nucleus through the fibers of the superior cerebellar peduncle. There are several routes over which these impulses may travel to reach the various motor systems and modify muscular movements. The first of these is the dentatorubrospinal path leading indirectly to lower motor neurons of the spinal cord. Fibers from the dentate nucleus (actually most of these fibers arise from the emboliform and globose nuclei) synapse with cells of the red nucleus which give rise to axons of the rubrospinal tract. This path crosses twice—once in the decussation of the superior cerebellar peduncle, and again in the rubrospinal tract near its origin—so that the origin and terminus are on the same side of the body. Another route traveled by efferent cerebellar impulses is the dentatothalamocortical path. Crossed fibers of the superior cerebellar peduncle which by-pass the red nucleus ascend to the ventral lateral nucleus of the thalamus. Thalamocortical fibers from this nucleus relay impulses to the motor area of the frontal lobe. It is clear that the cerebellum influences the activity of the pyramidal system through these circuits. Impulses to both facilitatory and inhibitory reticular nuclei are transmitted by the reticulospinal tracts to the motor neurons.

With respect to the efferent output of the cerebellar cortex, in general, the vermal cortex projects to the fastigial nucleus through corticonuclear fibers (that is Purkinje cell axons to the fastigial nucleus), the paravermal region projects to the emboliform and globose nuclei, and the lateral (hemisphere) region projects to the dentate nucleus. This is in keeping with the longitudinal zonal organization of the cerebellum.

Feed-Back Circuits Through the Cerebellum

The general scheme of operation of the cerebellum allows nerve impulses to be returned, or fed back, to the same region from which they originated. In this respect, cerebellar circuits are analogous to modern automatic control devices, or servomechanisms. The guided missile, for example, transmits radar signals which are picked up and fed to a mechanical computer. The computer, which may be thought of as analogous to the cortex of the cerebellum, detects any error in the missile's track and returns the proper radio messages to adjust its controls and put it back on course.

Briefly, the following are important feed-back circuits involving the cerebellum:

1. The vermal region receives information from the spinal cord and sends back information indirectly by the fastigial nucleus through the reticular formation (reticulospinal tracts) and vestibular nuclei (vestibulospinal tracts) to the cord.
2. The flocculonodular lobe receives information from the vestibular system and returns information through fastigiobulbar and fastigioreticulovestibular pathways.
3. The lateral (hemisphere) region receives information from the cerebral cortex and sends information back through the dentatothalamocortical path to exert an influence on the cerebrum and through the red nucleus to influence the spinal cord (rubrospinal tract).

CLINICAL SIGNS OF CEREBELLAR DYSFUNCTION

Disorders of the cerebellum, or of the fibers leading to and from the cerebellum, are accompanied by a number of characteristic signs, all of which concern the motor system:

A. *Ataxia*. Ataxia which is caused by cerebellar damage is manifested in several ways.

   1. Disturbances of posture and gait may be pronounced. Lesions of the midline region of the cerebellum cause difficulty in maintaining an upright stance. The loss of equilibrium is due to lack of muscle synergy and not to a defect in the pathway of conscious proprioception. Closing the eyes has very little worsening influence on this form of ataxia. The gait is staggering, not unlike that seen in drunkenness. A lesion located in one hemisphere of the cerebellum causes a tendency to fall toward the side of the lesion. If the patient attempts to walk in a straight line with the eyes closed, he may swerve to the side of the injured hemisphere.

   2. Decomposition of movement involves an action which requires the cooperative movement of several joints not properly coordinated, but is broken down into its component parts. For example, in bringing the hand to the mouth the joints of the shoulder, elbow, and wrist may be moved separately and not grouped together in one snychronized movement.

   3. Dysmetria is shown by the inability to stop a movement at the desired point. In reaching the hand toward an object, the patient either ·overshoots the goal or stops before it is reached. When he is asked to point his finger directly to the

finger of the examiner, the patient may instead point consistently to one side, a phenomenon known as past-pointing.

4. Dysdiadochokinesia, or adiadochokinesia, is the inability to stop one movement and follow it immediately by the directly opposite action. This is apparent on attempting to make rapid alternating movements of pronation and supination of the hands, or by tapping quickly with the fingers.

5. Scanning speech is due to asynergy of the muscles used in speaking. The spacing of sounds is irregular with pauses in the wrong places.

B. *Hypotonia.* The muscle tone is decreased which may be ascertained by palpation. The tendon reflexes are usually decreased on the side affected. A pendular knee jerk in which the leg swings freely back and forth several times is sometimes present.

C. *Asthenia.* The muscles which are affected by cerebellar lesions are weaker, and tire more easily than normal muscles.

D. *Tremor.* The tremor of cerebellar dysfunction is usually an intention tremor. It is evident during purposeful movements, but absent or diminished with rest. Lesions which are most apt to produce tremor are those that involve the efferent pathways of the superior cerebellar peduncle. The movements are coarse and arrhythmic.

E. *Nystagmus.* The nystagmus which is frequently present with cerebellar lesions may be accounted for by irritation of vestibular fibers in the cerebellum, or it may be due to the effect of pressure on the vestibular nuclei of the brain stem ventral to the cerebellum.

Cerebellar defects are compensated for, to a considerable extent, by other mechanisms of the brain if sufficient time is given. Consequently, symptoms are less severe in slowly progressing disease processes than in acute injuries of the cerebellum.

Somatotopical localization of separate body regions in the cerebellar cortex has been shown in experimental animals. It is important to note, however, that the right side of the body is under the influence of the right cerebellar hemisphere, and that any symptoms which occur unilaterally are found on the same side as the lesion in the cerebellum. *This contrasts strikingly with cerebral lesions which invariably produce contralateral effects.*

16
Lesions of the Brain Stem

Because of the compact arrangement of the structures of the brain stem, a single lesion nearly always damages several of them at once and produces a puzzling assortment of clinical signs. Logical interpretation of these effects depends on an understanding of the functional anatomy of fiber tracts and nuclei. The examples which follow illustrate some of the symptom complexes, or syndromes, associated with hemorrhages, vascular occlusions, tumors, or areas of degeneration in different parts of the brain stem. Many of these syndromes have been given eponyms, but since there is considerable lack of uniformity in their usage, only the more familiar ones will be named.

Lesions of the Basal Part of the Medulla

Several of the individual cranial nerves pass close to the lateral side of the pyramidal tract before they emerge from the brain stem. A single lesion that includes the nerve and the tract at this point produces nerve paralysis on the side of the lesion and contralateral *hemiplegia*, a condition referred to as *alternating hemiplegia*. For example, a lesion of the right hypoglossal nerve and the right pyramid results in left hemiplegia combined with paralysis of the muscles of the right half of the tongue (Fig. 34, lesion 1). The paralysis of the arm and leg is on the side opposite the lesion because the pyramidal tract subsequently crosses to the left. The usual signs of spasticity—increased muscle tonus, hyperreflexia, pathological re-

105

flexes and loss of superficial reflexes—will be present. The tongue deviates to the right side when protruded and, in time, the right half of the tongue will become atrophic.

An extension of this lesion across the midline may damage the left pyramid and produce additional signs of upper motor neuron involvement in the right extremities (Fig. 34, lesion 1a). If the same lesion is enlarged in the dorsal direction, it will affect the right medial lemniscus and there will be defects in tactile discrimination, muscle, joint and vibratory sense (Fig. 34, lesion 1b). Since the fibers of the medial lemiscus have been crossed previously in the lower part of the medulla, the sensory signs will appear on the left side of the body.

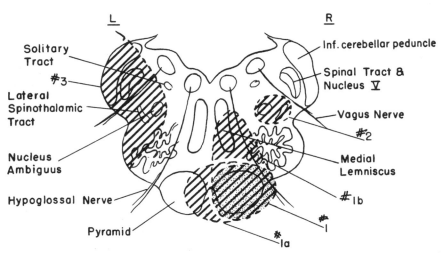

FIGURE 34. Cross section of the upper region of the medulla. The cross-hatched areas indicate positions of lesions: 1. Alternating hypoglossal hemiplegia. 1a. Same with extension across the midline to the opposite pyramid. 1b. Same with extension dorsally to include the medial lemniscus. 2. Lesion of the nucleus ambiguus and the lateral spinothalamic tract. 3. Lesion of the restiform body, spinal root and nucleus of nerve V, vagus nerve, and lateral spinothalamic tract. Syndrome of the posterior inferior cerebellar artery.

Lesions of the Central Region of the Upper Medulla

A small lesion in the lateral part of the reticular formation of the upper medulla may include the nucleus ambiguus and the lateral spinothalamic tract simultaneously (Fig. 34, lesion 2). When the lesion is on the right side, it causes a loss of pain and temperature sense on the left side of the body, except for the face. The sensory effects are contralateral because fibers of the lateral spinothalamic tract are crossed near their origin. Destruction of the nucleus ambiguus paralyzes the voluntary muscles supplied by the right vagus and glossopharyngeal nerves. Failure of the right side of the soft palate to contract causes difficulty in swallowing and, on phonation, the palate and uvula are drawn to the non-paralyzed left side. Loss of function of the right vocal cord lends to hoarseness of the voice.

A larger lesion in this region may extend to the medial lemniscus and to the solitary tract. Interrupting the fibers of the lemniscus causes the additional loss of proprioception and tactile discriminative sense on the left. Destruction of the solitary tract results in anesthesia of the mucosa of the right side of the pharynx and loss of taste sense on the right side of the tongue.

Lesions of the Dorsolateral Region of the Upper Medulla (Syndrome of the Posterior Inferior Cerebellar Artery)

The posterior inferior cerebellar artery, a branch of the vertebral artery, supplies the dorsolateral portion of the medulla. A lesion in this position is commonly the result of arterial occlusion by thrombosis. The damage involves the inferior cerebellar peduncle, the spinal tract and nucleus of the spinal tract, the lateral spinothalamic tract, the nucleus ambiguus, the vestibular nuclei, and the emerging fibers of the vagus and glossopharyngeal nerves (Fig. 34, lesion 3). Loss of function of the spinocerebellar tract results in cerebellar asynergia and hypotonia on the side of the lesion. Injury to the spinal tract of the trigeminal nerve blocks sensations of pain and temperature from that side of the face, while damage to the lateral spinothalamic tract is responsible for loss of pain and temperature sense in the limbs and trunk of the side opposite to the lesion. Because of its peculiar distribution, this sensory deficit has been called alternating analgesia. In addition to these features, the motor and sensory functions of the vagus and glossopharyngeal nerves are lost on the side of the injury, and there may be conjugate deviation of the eyes or nystagmus from irritation of the vestibular nuclei.

Lesions of the Basal Portion of the Caudal Part of the Pons

A lesion which is so placed that it includes the right pyramidal tract and the emerging fibers of the right abducens nerve results in alternating abducens hemiplegia (Fig. 35, lesion 1). There is an upper motor neuron type of paralysis of the left arm and leg as well as internal strabismus of the right eye. The tongue is usually not affected because the corticobulbar fibers to the hypoglossal nuclei run in the tegmentum and are not with the pyramidal tracts at this level.

Lesions of this part of the brain stem often extend far enough laterally to include fibers of the facial nerve and will also produce a peripheral type of facial paralysis. When the facial nerve is included, the condition is sometimes called *Millard-Gubler's syndrome* (Fig. 35, lesion 1a).

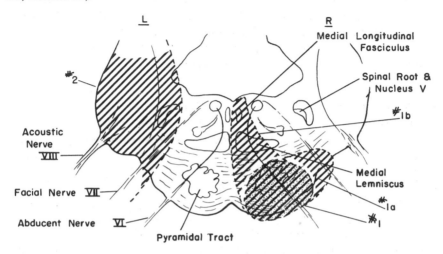

FIGURE 35. Cross section of the caudal region of the pons. The cross-hatched areas indicate positions of lesions. 1. Alternating abducent hemiplegia. 1a. Same with extension laterally to include the facial nerve. 1b. Same with extension dorsally to include the medial lemniscus and the medial longitudinal fasciculus. 2. Lesion of the lateral area of the pons including the acoustic nerve, cerebellar peduncles, facial nerve, spinal root and nucleus of nerve V, and lateral spinothalamic tract. Pontocerebellar angle syndrome.

A similar lesion with considerable dorsal expansion into the pontine tegmentum will involve the right medial lemniscus and the right medial longitudinal fasciculus (Fig. 35, lesion 1b). The effect of interrupting fibers of the medial lemniscus is loss of position and vibratory sense on the left side of the body. The corticomesencephalic tract, which has descended from the motor eye center of the left frontal lobe, has already crossed and is contained in the right medial longitudinal fasciculus. Cutting the tract at this point abolishes the ability to turn the eyes voluntarily to the right—*paralysis of right lateral gaze.* The eyes may be drawn to the left by the predominating influence of the non-paralyzed anagonistic muscles, but such an effect is temporary. The combination of symptoms produced by this lesion is known as the *syndrome of Foville.*

Lesions of the Pontocerebellar Angle

A slowly growing tumor which arises from Schwànn cells in the sheath of the acoustic nerve close to the attachment of the nerve to the brain stem exerts pressure on the lateral region of the caudal part of the pons near the pontocerebellar angle (Fig. 35, lesion 2). At first the symptoms are those of eighth nerve damage. There is progressive deafness, absence of normal labyrinthine responses and, sometimes, horizontal nystagmus. Later, cerebellar asynergia appears on the side of the lesion due to compression of the cerebellar peduncles. Damage to the spinal tract and nucleus of the fifth nerve abolishes the corneal reflex and causes diminished pain and temperature sensibility over the face on the side of the injury. A peripheral type of facial paralysis, also on the side of the lesion, results from the inclusion of fibers of the seventh nerve.

Lesions of the Middle Region of the Pons

A single lesion in the basal pàrt of the pons can affect the right pyramidal tract and the emerging fibers of the right trigeminal nerve to produce *alternating trigeminal hemiplegia* (Fig. 36, lesion 1).

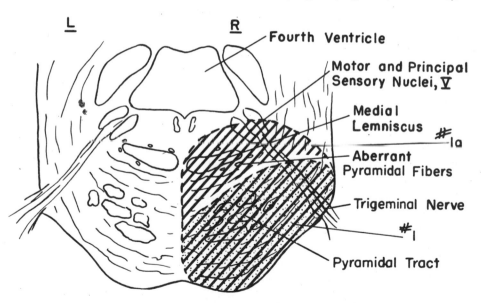

FIGURE 36. Cross section of the middle region of the pons. The cross-hatched areas indicate positions of lesions: 1. Alternating trigeminal hemiplegia. 2. Same with extension dorsally to include the medial lemniscus and aberrant pyramidal fibers.

There is spastic paralysis of the left arm and leg. The muscles of the right side of the jaw are paralyzed, and the chin deviates to the right. In addition, loss of the sensory fibers of the trigeminal nerve causes anesthesia of the right side of the face.

A lesion in the same region that extends deeper will enter the tegmentum of the pons and destroy the medial lemniscus. It also interrupts uncrossed fibers of the corticobulbar and corticomesencephalic tracts which have separated from the pyramidal tracts and, in this region, lie near the medial lemniscus (Fig. 36, lesion 1a). In addition to left hemiplegia, there is now a paralysis of the left half of the tongue, the left side of the soft palate, and of the superficial muscles of the lower part of the left side of the face due to interruption of upper neuron fibers to the motor nuclei of the seventh, ninth, tenth, and twelfth cranial nerves. The lesion also destroys the corticomesencephalic tract before it crosses, and blocks impulses from the right frontal lobe which produce voluntary turning of the eyes to the left. This results in *paralysis of left lateral gaze*. Damage to the right medial lemniscus is responsible for loss of conscious position sense and discriminative touch on the left side of the body.

Lesions of the Basal Part of the Midbrain (Weber's Syndrome)

A lesion of the right cerebral peduncle and the right oculomotor nerve produces spastic paralysis of the left arm and leg combined with external strabismus of the right eye and loss of the ability of raising the right upper eyelid. The right pupil is dilated because of interruption of the parasympathetic fibers in the third nerve. The corticobulbar tract may not be affected, since its fibers diverge from the pyramidal tract at this level and shift to a more dorsal position as they continue downward. However, if the lesion extends dorsally into the region of the substantia nigra, it may include most of these fibers and cause weakness of the tongue, soft palate and face contralateral to the lesion. In this instance, the tongue will deviate to the left, the soft palate and uvula will be drawn to the right, and there will be weakness of the muscles of the lower part of the left side of the face (Fig. 37, lesion 1).

Lesions of the Tegmentum of the Midbrain (Benedikt's Syndrome)

A lesion of the tegmentum of the midbrain affects the fibers of the oculomotor nerve, the medial lemniscus, the red nucleus and fibers

110

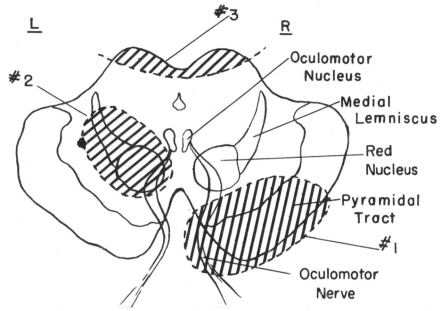

L R

#3

Oculomotor
Nucleus

#2

Medial
Lemniscus

Red
Nucleus

Pyramidal
Tract

#1

Oculomotor
Nerve

FIGURE 37. Cross section of the upper region of the midbrain. The cross-hatched areas indicate positions of lesions. 1. Alternating oculomotor hemiplegia (Weber's syndrome). 2. Lesion of the tegmentum including the medial lemiscus, the red nucleus, and fibers of the oculomotor nerve (Benedikt's syndrome). 3. Lesion of the tectum (Parinaud's syndrome).

of the superior cerebellar peduncle (Fig. 37, lesion 2). If the lesion is located on the left side, there is external strabismus and ptosis of the left eye from loss of the left oculomotor nerve. The right side of the body, including the face, shows a loss of tactile, muscle, joint, vibratory, pain and temperature sense from injury to the left medial lemniscus, which, at this level, has been joined on its lateral side by the spinothalamic tracts. Involvement of the red nucleus and the superior cerebellar peduncle, which contains efferent fibers from the right cerebellar hemisphere, produces tremor and irregular twitching movements of the right arm and leg.

Lesions of the Superior Colliculi (Parinaud's Syndrome)

Injury to the superior colliculi (Fig. 37, lesion 3) causes paralysis of upward gaze without affecting other eye movements. The anatomical basis for this is obscure, but experiments indicate that the area may contain a "center" for upward movement of the eyes. A pineal tumor could eventually cause this injury by pressure on the superior colliculi.

111

17
Vision

✓

For vision to occur, reflected rays of light from an object must strike the eye, be refracted by the cornea and lens, and form an image on the retina. The optic principles are the same as those of any camera and the image that is formed is upside down *(inverted)* and turned left for right *(reversed)*. The entire visual path within the brain is organized in a fashion which conforms with the peripheral optical system, so that the right hemisphere is presented with upside-down images of objects that lie to the left. This apparent distortion of position, however, is matched by other mechanisms of the brain. The motor areas of the frontal lobes, and the body-image contained in the somesthetic zones of the parietal lobe, are similarly inverted and reversed.

THE VISUAL PATHWAY

Light falling on the rods and cones of the retina, the first order neurons of the pathway, triggers a photochemical reaction in these cells. This initiates nerve impulses which are conducted to the cerebral cortex. The second neurons of the visual path are the bipolar cells within the retina. These cells synapse with ganglion cells (third-order neurons) of the retina whose axons converge toward the optic disc to form the *optic nerve* (n. II). Fibers from the macula, where visual acuity is sharpest, enter the temporal side of the optic disc. After perforating the scleral coat of the eye, the optic nerve fibers pass directly to the *optic chiasm* which is located at the anterior part of the sella turcica of the sphenoid bone immediately in front of the pituitary gland. A *partial decussation* takes place in the *chiasm. Fibers from the nasal halves of each retina cross; those from the temporal halves of each retina approach the chiasm and leave it without crossing* (Fig. 38). Optic fibers continue without any interruption behind the chiasm as two diverging optic tracts which go to the left and right geniculate bodies of the thalamus.

The fibers in front of the chiasm are designed as *optic nerves,* while those behind it are the *optic tracts.* Optic fibers terminate in the *lateral geniculate bodies,* superior colliculus, and pretectal area. Cells of the geniculate bodies give rise to fibers which form the *geniculocalcarine tract (optic radiation)* to the cortex of the occipital lobes. The radiation fibers are directed downward and forward at first. Then they bend backward in a sharp loop and form a flat band

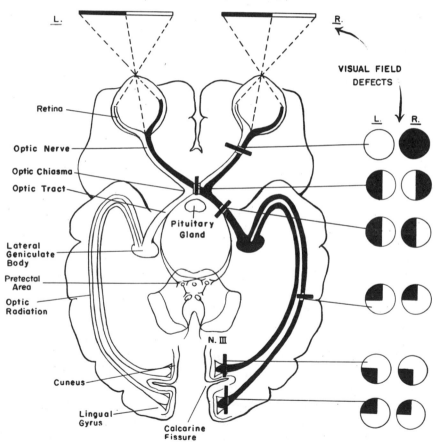

FIGURE 38. The visual pathway. On the right are maps of the visual fields with areas of blindness darkened to show the effects of injuries in various locations.

113

which passes through the temporal lobe, external to the inferior horn of the lateral ventricle, and sweeps posteriorly to the occipital lobe. The area of cortex that receives the optic radiation surrounds the *calcarine fissure* on the medial side of the occipital lobe. The *visual receptive area* (Brodmann's area 17) is also called the striate area because a cross section of the cortex contains a horizontal stripe (Gennari's line) which is visible to the naked eye. Areas 18 and 19, which adjoin area 17, are important regions for visual perception and for some visual reflexes, that is, visual fixation.

Effects of Lesions Interrupting the Visual Pathway

Destroying one optic nerve blinds the eye. Atrophy of the optic nerves affects some fibers but spares others, and instead of total blindness, there usually are areas of lost function in the peripheral part of the fields of vision of each eye.

The *visual fields* can be measured in detail with a perimeter, but a simpler way of examining them for gross defects is by the confrontation method. While the subject fixes his gaze straight ahead, an object is introduced from some point beyond the normal periphery of vision and moved slowly toward the line of vision. The point at which the object is first seen is noted, and after repeating the process in several directions, an estimate of the extent of the field of vision can be made. With optic atrophy there may be contraction of both visual fields, or a centrally located patch of visual loss *(scotoma)* may be found in each eye. Restricted visual fields, without any organic lesions, are encountered in some psychoneurotic patients to whom everything appears as if viewed through twin gun barrels. These patients, however, do not stumble over objects, and if there visual fields are accurately measured on repeated occasions, gross inconsistencies may be demonstrated.

A lesion of the optic tract behind the chiasm disconnects fibers from one half of each retina. If the right optic tract is destroyed, visual function is lost in the right halves of both retinae. *The result, however, is not described in terms of the retinae, but with reference to the disturbance that is produced in the visual fields.* In this instance there is blindness for objects in the left half of each field of vision, a condition known as left *homonymous hemianopia.* Even though one optic tract has been completely interrupted, vision is sometimes preserved in a small area at the fixation center, the area of the macula. Macular sparing cannot be explained anatomically, and opinions differ as to its significance. Lesions which destroy the entire visual area of the right occipital lobe, or all of the fibers of the right optic radiation, will also produce left homonymous hemianopia. Visual acuity of the parts of the retinae whose functions remain is not affected, and the patient may not be aware of the presence of hemianopia.

The *cuneus*, which is the gyrus above the calcarine fissure, receives visual impulses from the dorsal, or upper halves, of the retinae; the *lingual gyrus*, below the calcarine fissure, receives impulses that arise from the ventral, or lower halves. Thus a lesion that is confined to the right lingual gyrus cuts off visual impulses from the lower part of the right half of each retina. This produces a loss of vision in one quadrant, rather than hemianopia. Since the images which are focused on the lower part of the retina come from objects above the horizon line, there is, in this instance, an upper left quadrant defect (see Fig. 38). The visual impulses which go to the lingual gyrus travel in the ventral part of the optic radiation. Consequently, a lesion of the ventral fibers of the right optic radiation has the same effect as a lesion of the right lingual gyrus.

Lesions of the middle part of the optic chiasm are frequently produced by compression of these fibers from a tumor of the pituitary gland, or a craniopharyngioma which lies near the midline immediately behind the chiasm. The decussating fibers of the optic nerves are injured and visual impulses from the nasal halves of each retina are blocked. As a result, the left eye does not perceive images in the left half of its visual field, and the right eye does not record images in the right half of its field of vision. The defect is in the temporal field of each eye and is therefore called *heteronomous bitemporal hemianopia.*

18
Optic Reflexes

The Light Reflex

The constriction of the pupil which normally occurs when light is flashed into the eye constitutes the light reflex. The sensory receptors for this reflex are the rods and cones of the retina. The afferent pathway follows the course of the visual fibers of the optic nerve and tract as far as the lateral geniculate bodies, but instead of entering the geniculate body, the reflex fibers turn off in the direction of the superior colliculus (see Fig. 38). They end in a region rostral to the superior colliculus known as the *pretectal area.* Internuncial nerve cells located in this region send axons around the cerebral aqueduct to the Edinger-Westphal *nucleus,* a rostral subdivision of the oculomotor nucleus. The efferent path begins with cells in the Edinger-Westphal *nucleus* whose axons leave the midbrain in the oculomotor nerve and end in the *ciliary ganglion.* Postganglionic fibers coming from the ganglion enter the eyeball and supply the sphincter of the iris.

The response in the eye which is stimulated is the *direct reflex.* A *consensual light reflex* is shown by a similar, but weaker, constriction of the pupil of the other eye. The direct light reflex may be abolished by a lesion of the optic nerve, or by disease which damages the retina severely. Lesions of the visual path which are located caudal to the lateral geniculate bodies, however, do not interfere with the reflex fibers. In cortical blindness produced by a complete destruction of the primary visual areas of both occipital lobes, the light reflexes are preserved. The efferent path for the light reflex may be

116

interrupted by damage to the oculomotor nucleus, oculomotor nerve, or the ciliary ganglion. Neither a direct nor a consensual light reflex is then obtained in the affected eye.

Reflexes Associated with the Near-Point Reaction

When the eyes are directed to an object close at hand, three different reflex responses are brought into cooperative action.
1. Convergence. The medial recti muscles contract to move the eyes into alignment so that images in each eye focus on the same part of the retina. Otherwise the two images cannot be fused and diplopia will result.
2. Accommodation. The lenses are thickened as a result of tension by the ciliary muscles in order to maintain a sharply focused image.
3. Pupillary Constriction. The pupils are narrowed as an optical aid to regulate the depth of focus. The constriction does not depend on any change in illumination and is separate from the light reflex.

All three reactions may be initiated by voluntarily directing the gaze to a near object, but an involuntary (reflex) mechanism will accomplish the same results if an object is moved slowly toward the eyes.

The Argyll Robertson Pupil

One hundred years ago, Argyll Robertson described four cases of neurosyphilis in which the pupils failed to react to light but did constrict normally with accommodation. The sign later became a well-established clinical finding in syphilis of the central nervous system. Although the exact site of the lesions has never been proved, it is probably in the gray matter around the cerebral aqueduct. *Adie's pupil* is a benign condition characterized by a very weak light reflex which is delayed for several seconds and thus may be confused with the Argyll Robertson pupil.

The Visual Fixation Reflex

Voluntary mechanisms turn the head and eyes toward an object which occupies one's attention and will bring the desired image into approximately the same position on each retina. The final adjustments, which are necessary to produce identical correspondence of the two visual fields, are carried out by the fixation reflex. If the object is moving, this reflex also serves to hold it in view, involuntarily following its progress by causing appropriate turning movements of both eyes. The afferent pathway of the fixation reflex is from the retina to the visual cortex. The exact location and course of the efferent path is disputed, but it is certain that it begins in the cortex of the occipital lobe and goes to the superior colliculus or pretectum. Fibers arising from cells in the tectum reach the motor nuclei of cranial nerves III, IV, and VI by way of the medial longitudinal fasciculus. When the visual cortex receives images from the left and right retinae which do not match properly, impulses flow through the fibers of the occipitotectal tracts to bring the eyes into correct alignment for fixation.

The fixation is well demonstrated by a passenger who looks out of the window of a train at the passing scenery. His head and eyes turn slowly in the direction of apparent movement, then jump ahead quickly to fix the gaze on a new spot. This is done without awareness that the eyes are moving and is a true optokinetic reflex.

The fixation reflex is also used during the act of reading. Although we are unaware of it, the movement of the eyes along a line of print consists of several jerky movements (saccadic movements) with fixation pauses in between to allow visualization of a group of letters. These movements are not under voluntary control. Reading speed can be increased, however, by learning to take in more letters at once, or by making the pauses shorter. The difficulty of most slow readers does not lie in the oculomotor reflexes, but in the prolonged time required for each pause.

Protective Reflexes

An object which is quickly thrust in front of the eyes without warning causes a blink. This reflex response cannot be inhibited voluntarily. Afferent impulses from the retinae go to the tectum of the upper midbrain directly. From here, impulses are sent in the tectobulbar tracts to the nuclei of the facial nerves which activate the orbicularis oculi muscles and close the lids. A very strong stimulus, such as a sudden blinding flash of light, produces more extensive activity in the tectal region which sends impulses over tectospinal fibers as well as the tectobulbar tract. Besides closure of the eyes, there will be a "startle" response of the whole body musculature and the arms may be thrown upward across the face.

118

The Pain Reflex

Painful stimulation caused by pinching the skin, particularly at the neck, produces dilation of the pupils—the *ciliospinal reflex*. Although this reflex is well known, there are different versions of its pathway in the nervous system. Impulses which enter the spinal cord are said to stimulate sympathetic neurons whose axons ascend through the cervical sympathetic trunk to the dilator muscle fibers of the iris. On the other hand, it has been shown that the parasympathetic neurons of the Edinger-Westphal nucleus, which constrict the iris, are inhibited during the response.

Eye Movements

Eye movements are extremely complex and require the integrated effort of the cerebral cortex (occipital lobe and frontal eye fields), cerebellum, vestibular system, and reticular formation. All of these systems must converge on the oculomotor, trochlear, and abducens nuclei to control the extraocular muscles.

19

The Autonomic Nervous System

The autonomic nervous system, although a part of the peripheral nervous system, is the functional division which innervates *smooth and cardiac muscle* and the *glands* of the body. It consists of motor *(general visceral efferent)* fibers only; sensory fibers *(general visceral afferent)* which accompany the motor fibers to the viscera are not a part of the autonomic system. The autonomic nervous system functions at the subconscious level and is integrated with other body activites. The hypothalamus exerts the primary integrative influence on the autonomic system. Descending impulses from the brain stem and cerebral cortex, as well as local reflex stimuli, may govern the activity of the autonomic nervous system.

The autonomic nervous system is a two neuron chain. The cell bodies and their fibers are classified as follows:

1. The *preganglionic neuron* is the primary neuron which is located in the brain stem or cord (intermediolateral gray column in thoracic cord).

2. The *postganglionic neuron* is the postsynaptic or secondary neuron which is located in outlying ganglia and innervates the end organ. The postganglionic neurons outnumber the preganglionic neurons in an approximate ratio of 30 to 1.

DIVISIONS OF THE AUTONOMIC NERVOUS SYSTEM

The peripheral autonomic nerves (preganglionic fibers) have their origin from three regions in the brain and cord which provides an

120

anatomical basis for the two divisions of the autonomic nervous system. The *thoracolumbar outflow* consists of the fibers which arise in the *intermediolateral gray column* of the twelve thoracic and first lumbar segments of the spinal cord. This is the *sympathetic system.* The *cranial outflow* consists of fibers which arise in the Edinger-Westphal nucleus, superior and inferior salivatory nuclei and the dorsal motor nucleus of the vagus nerve. The *sacral outflow* consists of fibers which arise from cell bodies in the intermediate gray matter of *sacral segments two through four.* These fibers form the pelvic splanchnic nerves (nervi erigens). The cranial and sacral outflow share many anatomical and functional features and together form the *parasympathetic system.*

The autonomic system also has a physiological basis of division. The terminals of the parasympathetic postganglionic fibers liberate acetylcholine and are classified as *cholinergic.* With certain exceptions, notably those fibers which terminate in sweat glands, *norepinephrine*-like substances (sympathin) are released at the terminals of the sympathetic postganglionic fibers. The sympathetic system is classfied as *adrenergic.*

Many organs receive fibers from both the sympathetic and parasympathetic systems. When dual innervation occurs, the fibers frequently have opposing effects (for example, parasympathetic fibers to the stomach increase peristalsis and relax the sphincters while the sympathetic fibers have the opposite effect).

The Sympathetic Nervous System Division

The preganglionic fibers of the sympathetic system, which originate in the intermediolateral gray column, leave the spinal cord with the motor fibers of the ventral roots but soon separate from the spinal nerves to form the *white rami communicantes* which enter the *sympathetic trunks* (see Fig. 7). The latter are the paired ganglionated chains of nerve fibers which extend along either side of the vertebral column from the base of the skull to the coccyx. Some of the fibers of the white rami synapse with postganglionic neurons in the trunk ganglion *(paravertebral ganglion)* nearest their point of entrance. Other preganglionic fibers pass up or down the chain to end in paravertebral ganglia at higher or lower levels than the point of entrance.

Nonmyelinated, postganglionic fibers given off from the neurons in the sympathetic trunk ganglia form the *gray rami communicantes.* Each spinal nerve receives a gray ramus which is distributed to the blood vessels, arrector pili muscles, and sweat glands of the body wall throughout its dermatome. The gray rami outnumber the white since they are given off from the ganglia of the cervical, lower lumbar and sacral segments of the sympathetic trunk which do not have white rami.

The *cervical part* of the sympathetic trunk consists of ascending preganglionic fibers from the first four or five thoracic segments of the spinal cord. Three ganglia are present—*superior cervical, middle cervical,* and the *cervicothoracic* (stellate). The latter is formed by the fusion of the inferior cervical and first thoracic ganglia. In addition to providing gray rami for the cervical and upper thoracic spinal nerves, the cervical ganglia also give rise to *cardiac nerves* which enter the cardiac plexus to supply sympathetic innervation to the heart. The *carotid plexus* is derived from the superior cervical ganglion. This plexus follows the ramifications of the carotid arteries and furnishes the sympathetic innervation of the head. Some fibers end in blood vessels and sweat glands of the head and face; others supply the lacrimal and salivary glands. The eye receives sympathetic fibers which innervate the dilator muscles of the iris and the smooth muscle fibers of the eyelid.

The viscera of the abdominal and pelvic cavities are supplied by the splanchnic nerves. The *thoracic splanchnic nerves* (greater, lesser, and least) carry the preganglionic fibers from the levels of ganglia T5 to T12 to the *prevertebral ganglia* of the abdomen. The latter ganglia include the *celiac, superior mesenteric,* and *aorticorenal* which are located at the roots of the arteries arising from the dorsal aorta. The *lumbar splanchnic nerves* carry the preganglionic fibers from the levels of the upper lumbar ganglia. The lumbar splanchnics terminate in the *inferior mesenteric* and *hypogastric ganglia.* The postganglionic fibers from the prevertebral (collateral) ganglia form extensive plexuses which follow the ramifications of the visceral arteries to reach the organs of the abdomen and pelvis.

Injury to the cervical portion of the sympathetic system produces *Horner's syndrome.* The *pupil* of the injured side is constricted (miosis) because its dilator muscle is inactive. There is *mild ptosis* of the eyelid, but the lid can still be raised voluntarily. There is an apparent enophthalmosis. Absence of *sweating* (anhydrosis) and *vasodilation* on the affected side makes the skin of the face and neck appear reddened and it feels warmer and drier than the normal side. Horner's syndrome is commonly the result of a lesion of the cervicothoracic ganglion, or of the cervical part of the sympathetic chain. It also occurs when a lesion of the spinal cord destroys the preganglionic neurons at their origin in the eighth cervical and first thoracic segments (ciliospinal center). Lesions which involve the reticular formation of the brain stem or the upper cervical segments of the spinal cord may interrupt descending sympathetic pathways from the brain and cause a Horner's syndrome on the same side as the lesion.

Since the superficial blood vessels of the head dilate after sympathetic interruption, the cervicothoracic ganglion is sometimes injected with a local anesthetic in an effort to produce dilation of cerebral vessels and improve circulation after cerebral thrombosis. It is difficult to evaluate the effectiveness of stellate ganglion block because many patients improve whether they receive the treatment or not.

Sympathetic fibers are known vasoconstrictors and operations have been devised to increase the circulation by interrupting this innervation (sympathectomy). Lumbar sympathectomy, which is performed to increase the circulation in the lower extremity, is the most common procedure.

The Sympathetic Innervation of the Adrenal Gland

Stimulation of the sympathetic nervous system ordinarily produces generalized physiological responses rather than discrete localized effects. This is, in part, due to the wide dispersion of sympathetic fibers, but is augmented by the release of epinephrine from the adrenal glands which circulates in the blood and increases the effects of impulses in the postganglionic fibers. The medulla of the adrenal gland is supplied by preganglionic fibers (lesser and least splanchnic nerves) which end directly on the adrenal medullary cells without synapsing in an interposed ganglion. The cells themselves are derivatives of nerve tissue and, in effect, constitute a modified sympathetic ganglion. Pain, exposure to cold, and strong emotions such as rage and fear evoke sympathetic activity which mobilizes the body resources for violent action. Functions of the gastrointestinal tract are suspended and blood is shunted away from the splanchnic area. Heart rate and blood pressure are increased. The coronary arteries dilate. The bronchioles of the lung are dilated. Contractions of the spleen release extra red cells to the blood. This activity was described by Cannon as the "fight or flight" phenomenon.

The Parasympathetic Nervous System

The preganglionic fibers of the parasympathetic system are long and extend to the *terminal ganglia* located within (for example, the myenteric plexus) or very close to (for example, the ciliary ganglion)

123

the organs which they supply. The postganglionic fibers, as a result, are very short.

The *cranial division* of the parasympathetic system supplies the ciliary muscle and sphincter muscle of the iris through the oculomotor nerve and ciliary ganglion. Secretory preganglionic fibers from the nervus intermedius of the seventh cranial nerve synapse in the pterygopalatine and submandibular ganglia. Postganglionic fibers from the pterygopalatine ganglion innervate glands of the mucous membrane, nasal chamber and sinuses, palate and pharynx, and the lacrimal gland while the fibers of the submandibular ganglion supply the sublingual and submandibular glands. The otic ganglion, which receives preganglionic fibers of the ninth cranial nerve, supplies postganglionic fibers to the parotid gland. The vagus nerve supplies the preganglionic fibers to the heart, lungs, and abdominal viscera. The latter organs have the postganglionic neurons in associated plexuses adjacent to or within the walls of the viscus.

The sacral division, through the pelvic splanchnic nerves, supplies fibers to ganglia in the muscular coats of the urinary and reproductive tracts, colon (descending and sigmoid), and the rectum. In the pelvic region, the parasympathetic system is primarily concerned with mechanisms for emptying. Under strong emotional circumstances these fibers may discharge along with a generalized sympathetic response and produce involuntary emptying of the bladder and rectum. The parasympathetic fibers are responsible for penile erection. Stimulation by sympathetic fibers and not parasympathetic, initiates the contractions of the ductus deferens and seminal vesicles to produce ejaculation.

The Innervation of the Urinary Bladder

Motor control of the urinary bladder is primarily a parasympathetic function which, although purely reflex in infants, is brought under voluntary regulation in normal adults. The preganglionic fibers of the parasympathetic nerves to the bladder have their cell bodies in the intermediate region of the gray matter of sacral cord segments two, three, and four. They enter the pelvic spanchnic nerves and terminate on ganglia which are located in the wall of the bladder (Fig. 39). Short postganglionic fibers go to the detrusor muscle which guards the internal orifice of the urethra. Stimulation of the parasympathetic nerves of the bladder contracts the detrusor, relaxes the internal sphincter, and empties the bladder.

The *sympathetic* supply to the bladder originates in cells of the intermediolateral gray column of upper lumbar cord segments whose

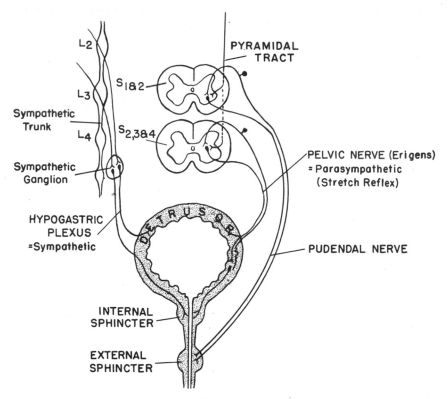

FIGURE 39. Autonomic innervation of the urinary bladder. The postganglionic parasympathetic ganglion cells are located in the pelvic plexus and the bladder wall.

axons pass through the sympathetic trunk to reach the inferior mesenteric ganglion by the lumbar splanchnic nerves. Post-ganglionic fibers continue to the wall of the bladder and to the internal sphincter. The functions of the sympathetic nerves are uncertain. They may assist the filling of the bladder by relaxing the detrusor muscle, but they have little influence on emptying mechanisms. Cutting the sympathetic nerves to the bladder does not seriously affect its function.

The external sphincter of the urethra is made up of striated muscle and innervated by regular motor fibers of the pudendal nerve along with other muscles of the perineum. The external sphincter may be closed voluntarily but relaxes by reflex action as soon as urine is released through the internal sphincter at the beginning of micturition.

The smooth muscle of the bladder responds to a stretch reflex operated by proprioceptors in its wall which send impulses to spinal cord segments sacral two, three, and four. The efferent reflex fibers return impulses over the pelvic splanchnic nerves to maintain tonus in the detrusor muscle while the bladder is filling. In the uninhibited bladder of infancy, and in some cases of mental deficiency or diffuse brain damage, the bladder fills nearly to its normal capacity, then a stronger reflex response takes place and it empties automatically. Voluntary suppression of urination is dependent on fibers that descend in the pyramidal tracts from the cortex of the paracentral lobules of the cerebrum. It is generally believed that these fibers exert an inhibitory effect on the detrusor reflex. The sensation of increased bladder tension and the desire to void are conveyed by sensory impulses in the afferent fibers of the pelvic nerves and ascending tracts of the spinal cord.

Lesions of the dorsal roots of sacral nerves, or of the posterior funiculi, which interrupt afferent reflex fibers produce an *atonic bladder*. The bladder wall is flaccid; its capacity greatly increased. Sensations of fullness of the bladder are entirely lost. As the bladder becomes distended there is incontinence and dribbling. Voluntary emptying is still possible, but it is incomplete and some urine is left in the bladder.

Injuries of the spinal cord cause a derangement of the bladder reflexes which usually results in contraction of sphincter muscles and retention of urine. Following transection of the spinal cord in the thoracic region an *automatic bladder* is frequently established. After several weeks, reflexes in the sacral segments of the cord may recover and begin to function. The bladder fills and empties spontaneously, or after the skin over the lower extremities is stimulated by scratching.

20
The Hypothalamus and Limbic System

DIENCEPHALON

The *diencephalon* is an ovid mass of gray matter situated deep in the brain rostral to the midbrain and ventral and caudal to the frontal lobes of the cerebrum. It is separated from the *basal ganglia* laterally by the fibers of the *internal capsule*. Ventrally, it extends from the *optic chiasma* to and including the *mammillary bodies*. The roof is formed by the *choroid plexus of the third ventricle*. The rostral limit may be demarcated by a line between the *interventricular foramen* and the optic chiasma. The caudal extent is demarcated by a line from the *pineal body* to the mammillary bodies. Except for a small area of fusion, the *massa intermedia* or *interthalamic adhesion*, the two halves of the diencephalon are separated by the slit-like cavity of the *third ventricle*. The diencephalon is divided into the following regions: thalamus, hypothalamus, subthalamus, and epithalamus.

Hypothalamus

The *hypothalamus* forms the floor and a part of the ventrolateral walls of the third ventricle. The shallow *hypothalamic sulcus* on the lateral walls of the third ventricle demarcates the hypothalamus from the thalamus.

The hypothalamus includes a number of well-defined structures. The *optic chiasm* is located at the rostral portion of the hypothalamic floor. The *tuber cinereum* is the portion of the hypothalamic floor between the optic chiasm and mammillary bodies. The *in-*

127

fundibulum (stalk of the pituitary) extends from the tuber cinereum to the pars nervosa of the hypophysis. The lumen of the third ventricle may evaginate into the infundibulum for a variable distance. The medial eminence is the portion of the hypothalamic floor between the optic chiasma and infundibulum. The *mammillary bodies* are paired, small, spherical masses located caudad to the tuber cinereum and rostral to the *posterior perforated substance.*

The hypothalamus may be subdivided into regions using the anatomical structures described as landmarks. The *supraoptic region* is the rostral area, the *mammillary region* is the caudal portion, and the *tuberal region* is the intervening portion.

Hypothalamic Nuclei

The hypothalamus consists of an admixture of neurons and fibers. The cells are somewhat aggregated and identified as nuclei. The more conspicuous nuclei will be identified in the three major regions. The following nuclei are found in the supraoptic region:
Supraoptic nucleus: straddles the lateral portions of the optic chiasma.
Paraventricular nucleus: is a group of cells dorsal to the supraoptic nucleus, in the lateral wall of the hypothalamus.
Preoptic nucleus: is the nuclear mass located between the supraoptic nucleus and the anterior commissure. Anatomically it is cerebral in location but it is hypothalamic functionally.
Several small nuclei are located in the tuberal region:
Dorsomedial nucleus: located in the dorsomedial portion of the lateral wall.
Ventromedial nucleus: located ventral to the dorsomedial nucleus.
Arcuate nucleus: located in floor of hypothalamus near infundibulum.
Lateral nucleus: located in floor of hypothalamus lateral to arcuate nucleus.
The following nuclei are located in the mammillary region:
Mammillary nuclei: are located within the mammillary bodies; usually subdivided into medial (larger) and lateral.
Posterior nucleus: located in the lateral wall of the hypothalamus dorsal to the mammillary nuclei.

Fiber Connections of the Hypothalamus

The fiber pathways of the hypothalamus are numerous and complex. Connections are not only made with the cerebrum, brain stem,

128

and cord but intrahypothalamic fibers also exist. A few pathways will be described.

The following pathways are afferent:

1. *Olfactohypothalamic* (in medial forebrain bundle): The fibers arise in the medial olfactory area and some synapse in the preoptic and lateral hypothalamic regions. The olfactovisceral and olfactosomatic functions are served by these fibers.

2. *Corticomammillary* (fornix): The fibers arise in the hippocampus and terminate in the mammillary bodies and possibly preoptic nuclei.

3. *Stria terminales:* This is a small fiber bundle, located in the terminal sulcus, which superficially demarcates the thalamus and caudate nucleus. The fibers extend from the amygdaloid nucleus to the preoptic and anterior hypothalamic nuclei, and to the ventromedial nucleus of the hypothalamus.

Additional afferent fibers arise in the thalamus and globus pallidus (thalamo- and pallidohypothalamic fibers). These are difficult to identify.

The following are some of the efferent pathways from the hypothalamus:

Fasciculus mammillaris princeps is the conspicuous bundle of fibers originating in the mammillary nuclei. It bifurcates to form:

1. *Mammillothalamic fasciculus*—terminates in the anterior thalamic nucleus.

2. *Mammillotegmental fasciculus*—terminates in the dorsal tegmental and interpeduncular nuclei of the midbrain.

3. *Dorsal longitudinal fasciculus*—located in the periventricular gray matter of the brain stem. The fibers connect the hypothalamus with the reticular formation of the midbrain and thence parasympathetic nuclei.

4. *Hypothalamo-hypophyseal tracts*—are the fibers which carry the neurosecretory material to the pars nervosa of the pituitary. The fibers take their origin in the supraoptic and paraventricular nuclei.

5. *Medial forebrain bundle*—fibers from the hypothalamic nuclei join the bundle as it continues toward the reticular formation of the midbrain.

Hypothalamus and Autonomic Nervous System

The hypothalamus has a regulatory influence on the autonomic nervous system. Stimulation of the *rostral portion* of the hypothalamus is excitatory to parasympathetic activity. It causes sweating, vasodilatation, and a decrease in the rate and force of the heart contraction. Lesions in this area allow sympathetic effects to have precedence which may result in increased cardiac activity, hyperthermia (fever), and panting. Stimulation of the *caudal portion* of the hypothalamus causes an excitation of the sympathetic system. The rate and force of the heart contractions are increased, vasoeonstriction occurs, respiration is increased, dilatation of the pupil occurs, and peristalsis is inhibited. One effect of a lesion in this area is the production of a hypothermic animal.

Hypothalamic Pituitary Relationships

The tubules of the kidney are under the influence of an antidiuretic hormone (ADH) secreted by the pars nervosa of the hypophysis for the reabsorption of large amounts of water from the glomerular filtrate. *Diabetes insipidus*, caused by a deficiency in ADH, is characterized by an excessive urinary output (polyuria) accompanied by excessive thirst (polydipsia). The axons of the neurons located in the supraoptic and paraventricular nuclei carry neurosecretory droplets in the hypothalamohypophyseal tract to be released in the pars nervosa. The Herring bodies, seen in the pars nervosa, are believed to represent the stored secretion. It has not been determined whether the neurosecretion is the hormone or whether the polypeptide is modified by the cells of the pars nervosa. This region of the hypothalamus functions as an osmoreceptor and is sensitive to the salt content of the fluids which bathe the supraoptic and paraventricular nuclei. If the sodium chloride level is high, more neurosecretion is elaborated and released to facilitate additional water reabsorption by the kidney tubules. It is believed that the supraoptic nucleus is correlated with the release of ADH and the paraventricular nucleus is correlated with the hormone oxytocin.

There is also evidence that the hypothalamus influences the secretory activity of the pituitary pars distalis. No connecting fibers are present, but a vascular link is established by the *hypophyseal portal system* which is a network of venous capillaries which conveys the neurohumoral substance from the infundibular region and medial eminence to the pars distalis. The so-called "releasing factor" for ovulation has its origin in the medial eminence. The hypothalamus may also affect the secretion of the "trophic hormones" by the pars distalis. The precocious development of puberty which occurs in association with hypothalamic tumors may be the result of excessive gonadotrophin caused by an excess of neurosecretory material.

Hypothalamic Centers and Appetite

The tuberal region has nuclei which are correlated with the feeding response. The *ventromedial nucleus* is designated as the "satiety center" while the *lateral nucleus* is the "feeding center." Small lesions in the ventromedial region of the hypothalamus cause experimental animals to eat voraciously. If permitted, they consume more food than they need and soon become fat. A lesion placed in the region of the lateral nucleus abolishes the appetite and leads to weight loss and emaciation. The Fröhlich, or adiposogenital, syndrome is characterized by underdevelopment of the gonads and obesity. It has been associated with a lesion in the tuberal region of the hypothalamus.

Regulation of Body Temperature

The anterior, or rostral, part of the hypothalamus plays an important role in temperature regulation by participating in mechanisms which dissipate excess body heat. When temperature of the blood rises, cells in this region send impulses over descending fibers to produce sweating and to cause dilation of the blood vessels of the skin which lowers the temperature. Cells located in the posterior part of the hypothalamus act to increase the heat of the body and prevent its loss. Fibers descending to the spinal cord constrict the vessels of the skin. At the same time sweating is inhibited and there may be shivering in which the somatic muscles generate heat.

Injury to the anterior part of the hypothalamus, as for example by surgery in that region, may impair the ability to dissipate heat and result in hyperthermia which is known as "neurogenic fever."

The Hypothalamus and Emotion

It is clear that the hypothalamus dispatches the autonomic discharge of nerve impulses that produce the physical expression of emotion: acceleration of the heart rate, elevation of blood pressure, flushing (or pallor) of the skin, sweating, goosepimpling of the skin, dryness of the mouth, and disturbances of the gastrointestinal tract. However, emotional experience includes subjective aspects or "feelings" which are assumed to involve the cerebral cortex. Furthermore, mental processes in the cortex which possess strong emotional content are fully capable of bringing forth hypothalamic reactions. Pathways which connect the cerebral cortex and the hypothalamus

are therefore considered to play an intimate **part** in the mechanisms of emotion.

Conduction pathways between the hypothalamus and the cortex are diverse and, in some instances, circuitous. They are concerned with the most primitive part of the forebrain, the rhinencephalon, which was formerly regarded as having primarily olfactory functions.

The major afferent connection of the hypothalamus is the *fornix,* a conspicuous tract ending in the *mammillary nuclei.* The fornix arises from the *hippocampus,* which is formed by an infolding of the inferior surface of the temporal lobe along the line of the hippocampal fissure. Fibers of the fornix proceed backward on the ventricular surface of the hippocampus, then arch forward under the corpus callosum. The fornix completes its nearly ring-shaped course by turning downward and back to reach the mammillary body (Fig. 40). The efferent connection of the mammillary body is the *mammillothalamic tract,* a prominent bundle of fibers passing directly to the

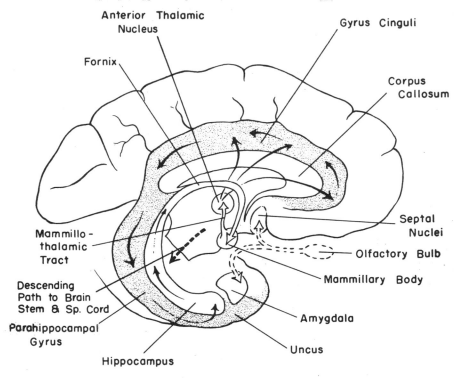

FIGURE 40. Main connections between the hypothalamus and the cerebral cortex. The limbic lobe is shaded. Solid arrows show the hypothetical circulation of impulses during the experiencing of emotion. The thick dotted arrow indicates the descending path to the brain stem and spinal cord for expressing emotion. Olfactory afferent fibers are lightly dotted.

132

anterior nucleus of the thalamus. The anterior thalamic nucleus sends fibers to the *cingulate gyrus,* which is the long gyrus next to the corpus callosum on the medial aspect of the cerebrum. The cingulate gyrus encircles the corpus callosum and, in its posterior part, is continuous through a narrowed strip (the isthmus) with the *parahippocampal gyrus,* the most medial convolution of the temporal lobe. Together the cingulate gyrus, isthmus, parahippocampal gyrus, and the uncus, an eminence near the front of the hippocampal gyrus form a ring of cortex known as the *limbic lobe* of the brain (see Fig. 40).

It has been suggested by Papez that the hippocampus, fornix, mammillothalamic tract, and anterior thalamic nucleus form part of a circuit by which impulses are transferred from the hypothalamus to the cortex and returned by the cortex to the hypothalamus. According to this theory, hypothalamic stimuli are projected to the cingulate gyrus by way of the anterior nucleus of the thalamus. Association fibers from the cingulate gyrus transmit this activity to other areas of the cortex and produce the emotional coloring of thought which is experienced subjectively during the expression of emotion. The reverse side of the circuit is offered to explain how emotional display is produced by psychic activity. Impulses are funneled through the cingulate gyrus and isthmus to the parahippocampal gyrus. Short fibers connect the parahippocampal gyrus with the hippocampus which lies beside it, but buried from sight. Fornix fibers to the mammillary bodies then carry the excitation to the hypothalamus which activates the peripheral autonomic nervous system. If this enter circuit is a reverberatory one, it may be possible for impulses to circulate continually and, by reinforcement, cause an emotional experience to be intensified.

Among the symptoms produced by the removal of both temporal lobes in humans is an attitude of indifference and a total loss of emotional responses. The operation removes a part of the hippocampus and interrupts the corticohypothalamic circuits. While this offers some tentative support, the Papez theory has, so far, remained largely speculative. It has been demonstrated in monkeys (Klüver-Bucy syndrome) that when the rostral part of the temporal lobe is removed, aggressive animals become tame, docile animals become bold, and additionally, some exhibit hypersexual behavior. It has also been suggested that the limbic system plays a role in memory. In man, where there is evidence of bilateral lesions in the hippocampus and amygdaloid nuclear complexes, long-term memory is retained but recent memory is impaired (Korsakoff's syndrome).

21

The Thalamus

The thalamus comprises the dorsal portion of the diencephalon. The relation to the hypothalamus and subthalamus has been described previously. The thalamus is bounded medially by the wall of the third ventricle and laterally by the posterior limb of the internal capsule. The dorsal surface of the thalamus has been covered by the overgrowth of the forebrain, and the roof of the thalamus is the chorioid plexus of the third ventricle. A groove, the *terminal sulcus*, which contains the *stria terminalis*, a longitudinal band of fibers, and the *vena terminalis*, demarcates the thalamus from the caudate nucleus along the dorsolateral margin.

The dorsal portion of the thalamus is subdivided into unequal thirds by the *internal medullary lamina*. This band of myelinated fibers demarcates the medial and lateral nuclear masses (Fig. 41). The lamina bifurcates at its rostral extent to encompass the anterior nucleus. The centromedian nucleus is enclosed within the medullary lamina in the center of the thalamus.

The thalamus serves as the station from which, after synaptic interruption, impulses of all types are relayed to the cerebral cortex. Processes of correlation and integration occur within the thalamus but conscious interpretation of peripheral sensory stimuli, except for pain, is not considered to occur at this level. The thalamus may be concerned with focusing the attention, perhaps by temporarily making certain cortical sensory areas especially receptive and other less receptive.

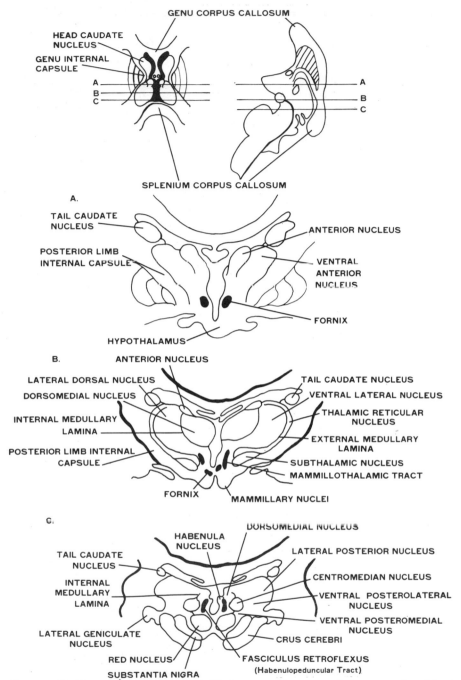

FIGURE 41. Transverse sections (A,B,C) depicting the major thalamic nuclei. The outline drawings of a horizontal section and a midsagittal brain stem preparation indicate the levels of the individual figures (A,B,C).

Thalamic Nuclei and Their Connections

I. *Medial Nuclear Mass* (located medial to the internal medullary lamina) contains one major nucleus, the *dorsomedial nucleus (DM)*, which is subdivided into *small cell (parvocellular)* and *large cell (magnocellular)* components. The small cell portion has a large reciprocal relationship with most of the frontal lobe (prefrontal cortex, areas 9, 10, 11, and 12) and is involved in emotional expression and behavior. The large cell component is interrelated with the hypothalamus, amygdala, and the orbital portion of the frontal lobe. The DM nucleus has many interconnections with other thalamic nuclei including the intralaminar and midline nuclei, and the lateral thalamic nuclear mass.

II. *Lateral Nuclear Mass* (located lateral to the internal medullary lamina) is subdivided into a *dorsal tier of nuclei* and a *ventral tier of nuclei:*

A. *Dorsal tier of nuclei* include, in a rostrocaudal direction
1. *lateral dorsal nucleus (LD)*— can be considered as the caudal extension of the anterior thalamic nucleus (A) and interconnects with the cingulate gyrus, precuneus, and mammillary bodies.
2. *lateral posterior nucleus (LP)*— is reciprocally connected with the caudal aspect of precuneus and with the superior parietal lobule (areas 5 and 7). It receives input from the medial and lateral geniculate bodies (MG and LG) and from the ventral posterior nuclear complex (VP).
3. *pulvinar (P)*— is the large posterolateral projection of the thalamus and connects reciprocally with a large association area of the parietal, temporal, and occipital cerebral cortex. Similar to the LP nucleus, it receives input from the MG, LG, and VP nuclei of the thalamus.

B. *Ventral tier of nuclei* include, in a rostrocaudal direction
1. *ventral anterior nucleus (VA)*— is subdivided into *small* and *large cell* populations. The large cell component receives its input from the substantia nigra (SN) and the small cell portion receives fibers from the medial aspect of the globus pallidus (GP). The VA nucleus also receives fibers from other thalamic nuclei (intralaminar and midline), the brain stem reticular formation, and the cerebral cortex. It projects to the caudate nucleus and the premotor cortex (primarily area 6 which includes the *supplementary motor zone* located on the medial aspect of the superior frontal gyrus immediately rostral to area 4.)

136

2. *ventral lateral nucleus (VL)*—is similar to the VA nucleus in that it contains both *small and large cell components* which receive fibers from the GP and SN respectively, and it receives fibers from other thalamic nuclei, the brain stem reticular formation, and the cerebral cortex. It differs from the VA nucleus in that it receives a major input from the cerebellum *(dentatothalamic tract)*, a minor input from the red nucleus *(rubrothalamic tract)*, and is reciprocally related to the *precentral gyrus*, area 4, the *primary motor region* of the cerebral cortex.
3. *ventral posterior nuclear complex (VP)*—is referred to as the *ventrobasal complex* by physiologists, and consists of two major subdivisions, the *ventral posteromedial nucleus (VPM)*, which is also called the semilunar or arcuate nucleus, and the *ventral posterolateral nucleus (VPL)*. Some authorities include a third, smaller component, the ventral posterointermediate nucleus (VPI) which is sandwiched in between the VPL and VPM nuclei.

   The VP nuclear complex is the main sensory region of the thalamus. Much of the information processed in this complex is both place and modality specific with small receptive fields. It is a synaptic station for the medial lemniscus, gustatory paths, secondary trigeminal tracts, and part of the spinothalamic system. The sensory tracts from the face terminate in the VPM nucleus while those from the remainder of the body synapse in the VPL nucleus. Consequently, it is *somatotopically organized* such that the input from the lower portion of the body is most laterally represented and that from the upper part most medially. This nuclear complex projects primarily to the *postcentral gyrus*, areas 3, 2, and 1, the *primary somesthetic cortex*. The postcentral gyrus is somatotopically organized such that the face is represented ventrolaterally (thus receiving the projection from VPM), and the leg dorsomedially (receiving its input from VPL). The cells in this region are both modality and place specific so that the various sensory inputs can be discreetly localized. The VP nuclear complex also projects to the *secondary somesthetic cortex* which is located in the most ventral aspect of the precentral gyrus (superior lip of the lateral cerebral fissure) and extends caudally to some extent in the parietal lobe.
4. *posterior nuclear group (PO)*—is a region of the thalamus located just caudal to the VP complex, medial to the

medial geniculate body (MG), and ventral to the pulvinar (P). It receives a *bilateral input from the spinothalamic tracts and is not somatotopically organized.* It contains large, diffuse receptive fields. Other sensory modalities also project to this nucleus. The PO complex projects primarily to the *secondary somesthetic cortex.*

5. *metathalamic nuclei*—include the medial (MG) and lateral (LG) geniculate bodies:

   (a) *medial geniculate body (MG)*—lies adjacent to the superior colliculus and receives bilateral auditory impulses from the nucleus of the inferior colliculus (IC) through the brachium of the IC. It projects, through the auditory radiations, to the auditory cortex of the superior temporal gyrus, specifically to the transverse gyrus of Heschl, area 41.

   (b) *lateral geniculate body (LG)*—the main portion of this nuclear complex in man contains 6 layers and receives fibers from both eyes. It is *reciprocally connected* via the optic radiations (geniculocalcarine tract) to the visual cortex of the occipital lobe, area 17. It is also interconnected to the pulvinar and possibly other thalamic nuclei.

III. *Anterior Nucleus (A)* is actually a complex of three nuclei located in the conspicuous anterior tubercle of the thalamus. This nucleus, in which the mammillothalamic tract terminates, has reciprocal connections with the cingulate gyrus and the hypothalamus. This is an important relay nucleus in the *limbic system.*

IV. *Intralaminar Nuclei* are numerous small, diffuse collections of nerve cells within the internal medullary lamina. In the caudal aspect of the lamina there are two more circumscribed intralaminar nuclei that can be delineated, the *centromedian nucleus (CM)*, which lies adjacent to the VP complex, and the *parafascicular nucleus (PF)*, which is located immediately medial to the CM nucleus.

In general, the intralaminar nuclei represent the rostral extent of the ascending *reticular system.* They *project diffusely to the entire neocortex*, are interconnected with other thalamic nuclei, and receive *bilateral input from the spinothalamic system.* The CM nucleus receives fibers from the globus pallidus (GP) and area 4 of the cerebrum and, in conjunction with the PF nucleus, projects to the putamen and possibly caudate nucleus. The PF nucleus receives fibers from area 6 of the cerebrum.

V. *Midline Nuclei* are very diffuse, small nuclei located in the periventricular region and in the interthalamic adhesion. Most likely, they are involved in the regulation of visceral phenomena and are interconnected with the dorsomedial nucleus (DM) and the hypothalamus.

VI. *(Thalamic) Reticular Nucleus* is a thin layer of cells sandwiched between the posterior limb of the internal capsule and the external medullary lamina. It is actually a *derivative of the ventral thalamus.* There is disagreement as to whether or not this nucleus should be considered part of the reticular system. It *does not project fibers to the cerebral cortex,* instead it sends fibers to thalamic nuclei, brain stem reticular formation, and to other parts of the thalamic reticular nucleus. It does receive fibers from the cerebrum. It should be noted that nearly all thalamic efferent projections to the cortex must pass through, and possibly influence, this nuclear complex. Consequently, its circuitry is structured such that it may play a major, yet poorly understood, role in the regulation of thalamic activity. The feedback of the cerebral cortex to this nucleus may provide a mechanism whereby the cerebrum can selectively screen the information that it receives.

Functional Categorization of Thalamic Nuclei

Classically, the thalamic nuclei have been categorized as being either specific or nonspecific. This nomenclature is confusing particularly in the case of the term nonspecific for it has also been considered to mean diffuse, association, and/or subcortical. Although there is still not complete agreement with respect to the terminology and function of the various thalamic nuclear groups, the terms employed by the leading authorities will be used in this discussion.

1. *Specific Nuclei* are those nuclei which have reciprocal relations with specific areas of the cerebrum known to have specific sensory or motor functions. They receive an input from the ascending pathways or major relay nuclei and include most of the *ventral tier nuclei* of the lateral nuclear mass: the LG, MG (some authorities do not consider the anterior nucleus in the specific category but rather in the association nuclei), VA (in part), VL, and VP nuclei.

2. *Association Nuclei* are those nuclei which do not receive direct input from ascending tracts. They have reciprocal connections with the association areas of the cerebral cortex. The main nuclei included are the *dorsal tier nuclei* in the lateral nuclear

mass, namely, the LD, LP, and pulvinar. A portion (parvocellu-lar) of the DM nucleus is also included.

3. *Subcortical Nuclei* have neither direct afferent or efferent connections with the cerebral cortex and include: the DM (in part), VA (in part), intralaminar, and thalamic reticular nuclei.

EPITHALAMUS

The epithalamus is the most dorsal division of the diencephalon. It is the only roof portion of the diencephalon consisting of nervous tissue. The major structures of this region are the pineal body (epiphysis), the habenular nuclei and commissure, the posterior commissure, the striae medullares, and the roof of the third ventricle.

The *pineal body* is the dorsal diverticulum of the diencephalon. It is a cone-shaped structure which projects backward over the tectum of the midbrain. Microscopically, it consists of glial cells (astrocytes), and parenchymal cells (pinealocytes). No neurons are present but there is an abundance of nerve fibers. Calcareous accumulations (corpora arenacea) are conspicuous features of the pineal body after middle age. The function of the epiphysis has been a controversial subject. At present, it is believed to have a secretory role which is associated with development and growth.

The *habenular nuclei* are located in the dorsal margin of the base of the pineal body. The afferent fibers to the habenula have their origin in the septal and olfactory nuclei and lateral hypothalamus and are carried in the *stria medullaris*. The stria medullaris forms a small ridge on the dorsomedial margin of the thalamus. The efferent fibers of the habenula, the *habenulopeduncular tract* or fasciculus retroflexus, is a conspicuous, dense bundle of fibers which terminates in the interpeduncular nucleus. Fibers from the latter nucleus descend to synapse in the motor nuclei of some cranial nerves. Hence the habenula appears to be a relay nucleus for olfactory impulses which regulate a primitive reflex (food getting).

The *habenular commissure* consists of stria medullaris fibers crossing over to the contralateral habenular nuclei. The *posterior commissure*, located ventral to the base of the pineal body, carries decussating fibers of the superior colliculi or tectum (visual reflex) and possibly fibers from other sources.

22

Rhinencephalon and Olfactory Reflexes

The rhinencephalon, which consists of the olfactory nerves, bulbs, tracts and striae, paraolfactory area (subcallosal region), anterior perforated substance, and the prepyriform region, is relatively prominent in the brain of macrosmatic vertebrates. As vision is utilized more exclusively, dependence on the olfactory sense decreases. The vertebrates utilizing vision more exclusively are classified as microsmatic; the human being is an example.

Peripheral Olfactory Apparatus

The peripheral olfactory receptors are found in specialized areas of the nasal mucosa designated as the *olfactory epithelium*. In man, the latter, generally pseudostratified columnar epithelium in type, is located on the superior concha, the roof of the nasal chamber and on the upper portion of the nasal septum. The receptor cells have elongated proximal processes which, grouped as filaments, pass through the fenestra of the cribriform plate as the olfactory nerve. The olfactory nerves pierce the surface of the olfactory bulb to synapse with neurons in the rostral portion.

Olfactory Bulbs and Olfactory Striae

The olfactory bulbs rest on the cribriform plate. The so-called laminar architecture of the bulb is difficult to demonstrate in the human being. The rostral portion of the bulb contains three types of second order neurons:

1. *Mitral cells* are the larger, triangular cells which may synapse with a number of olfactory fila, tufted cells, and/or granule cells.
2. *Tufted cells* are smaller and more peripheral than mitral cells. They synapse with olfactory fila in a bushy-like synapse known as the olfactory glomerulus. The olfactory glomerulus also appears at the synapse of the olfactory fila with the mitral cells.
3. *Granule cells* are the smallest neurons of the bulb which serve an inhibition function. The anterior olfactory nucleus, in the caudal portion of the olfactory bulb, consists of a number of groups of neurons. It contains the cells of origin of the olfactory portion of the anterior commissure.

The paired olfactory tracts, which are narrowed caudal continuations of the olfactory bulbs, lie in the olfactory sulcus. The tract soon bifurcates into medial and lateral striae. Some of the fibers of the medial olfactory stria enter the subcallosal area and then the rostral portion of the anterior commissure to be returned to the opposite olfactory bulb. The remainder of the fibers, which terminate in the olfactory trigone within the anterior perforated substance, are believed to be mitral cell processes.

The lateral stria, composed of mitral cell processes primarily, skirt the lateral margin of the anterior perforated substance to reach the prepyriform cortex in the region of the uncus. The primary olfactory cortex is considered to be the region in which the lateral olfactory stria terminate. Some fibers from this area are projected to area 28 (parahippocampal gyrus) which is known as the secondary cortical area. The olfactory system is the only sensory system which sends direct impulses to the cortex without the utilization of the thalamus as a relay center.

Olfactory Reflexes

The olfactory reflex connections are numerous and complex. The following three pathways are described in their simplest form. The fact that reciprocal connections may be present is recognized but omitted for the sake of clarity.

Fibers arising, directly or indirectly, from the three terminal regions of the olfactory striae are conveyed caudally over the stria medullaris to synapse primarily with the dorsomedial nucleus of the thalmus; a few fibers synapse with neurons in the habenular nucleus. The latter nuclei are located at the base of the pineal body in the epithalamus. Fibers arising in the habenular nucleus, the habenu-lopeduncular tract, arch ventrally to terminate in the interpeduncular nucleus. Fibers extend from here to the reticular nuclei in the tegmentum which sends out fibers that are carried by the dorsal longitudinal fasciculus to brain stem nuclei (superior and inferior salivatory nuclei and dorsal motor nucleus of the vagus).

The most primitive pathway involves fibers arising in the terminal areas of the olfactory cortex which are conveyed indirectly to the reticular formation via the medial forebrain bundle. Various cranial nerve nuclei may then synapse with fibers that originated in the reticular formation.

The following circuit probably enables one to determine whether an odor is pleasant or unpleasant. This pathway follows that of the limbic system which has been described previously. Fibers from the uncus extend to the secondary cortex in the parahippocampal gyrus. Association fibers connect the latter to the hippocampus and fibers from this area are carried over the fornix to the mammillary bodies. The fibers of the mammillothalamic tract* synapse in the anterior nucleus of the thalamus. Thalamic projections are conveyed to the cingulate gyrus which then sends association fibers into the cerebral cortex of the frontal lobes (Fig. 42).

Clinical Importance

Anosmia may be caused by a number of factors. The most frequent is the common cold. Other factors may be: nasal irritants, fracture of the ethmoid bone, certain drug intoxications, meningitis, psychoses, and association with uncinate fits. Hyperosmia may occur in some hysterias and has been observed following drug addiction.

It also will be remembered that the subarachnoid space is in close approximation to the olfactory mucosa. This area is sometimes implicated in infections.

---

*It will be recalled that the fasciculus mamillaris princeps, which arises in the mammillary bodies, splits into the mammillothalamic and the mammillotegmental tracts. The later, as a consequence, could convey impulses to the tegmentum which could also stimulate motor nuclei.

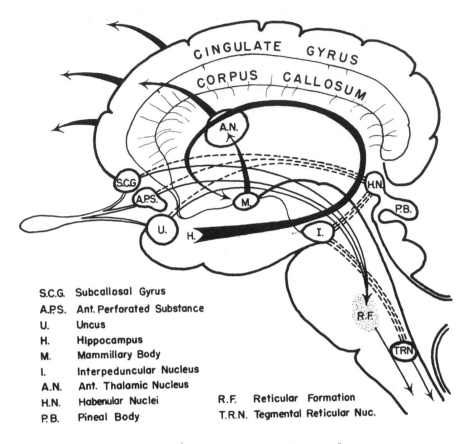

S.C.G. Subcallosal Gyrus
A.P.S. Ant. Perforated Substance
U.   Uncus
H.   Hippocampus
M.   Mammillary Body
I.   Interpeduncular Nucleus
A.N.   Ant. Thalamic Nucleus
H.N.   Habenular Nuclei   R.F.   Reticular Formation
P.B.   Pineal Body   T.R.N. Tegmental Reticular Nuc.

FIGURE 42. Diagram indicating olfactory reflexes.

23

The Cerebral Cortex

In popular opinion the cerebral cortex is thought of as the site of the mind and the intellect. Sherrington visualizes it dramatically as "... an enchanted loom where millions of flashing shuttles weave a dissolving pattern...." Scientific thought considers it to be the area which carries out a final integration of neural mechanisms. These and other similar generalizations reveal the incompleteness of our true understanding of cortical mechanisms. The direct evidence that is available of the functions of the cerebral cortex in humans comes from three principal sources: (1) from the study of localized destructive lesions and surgical removals; (2) from the sensations and physical responses of conscious patients when electrical stimulation is deliberately applied to different points on the surface of cortex (Fig. 43; and (3) from the patterns of response in epileptic seizures which arise from an irritative lesion in one part of the cortex.

NEURONS OF THE CEREBRAL CORTEX

The convoluted surface of the cerebral hemispheres contains a mantle of gray matter, thickly studded with cells which are arranged in layers. The *isocortex* (neocortex), which comprises about 90 per cent of the cerebral surface, contains six layers of cells while the *allocortex* contains three. The allocortex includes the *paleocortex* (olfactory cortex), and the *archicortex* (hippocampus and dentate gyrus). A third region of the cerebral surface, the *mesocortex* (including the cingulate gyrus and part of the parahippocampal gyrus),

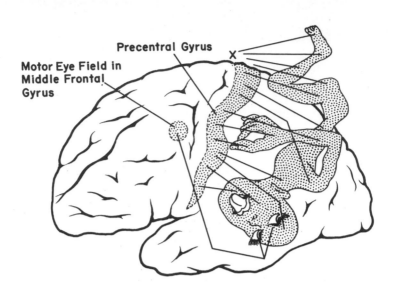

Motor Eye Field in Middle Frontal Gyrus

Precentral Gyrus

X

FIGURE 43. Manikin illustrating the topographic representation of the right side of the body in the motor area of the left frontal lobe.

contains between three and six layers depending upon the location. From the surface, the layers of the neocortex have been named: I *molecular;* II *external granular;* III *external pyramidal;* IV *internal granular;* V *internal pyramidal;* and VI *multiform.* In general, afferents to the cortex synapse in layers I through IV, while efferents arise from layers V and VI. Besides the horizontal laminations, the cells of the cortex are loosely organized into vertical columns with radial fibers interspersed between them. *The vertical columns are extremely important and considered to be the functional units of the cortex.* Short axons make connections within the columns to form a great variety of closed chains, or loops. Some of the fibers which terminate on the cells of the cortex cone from the thalamus *(projection fibers)* primarily to layer IV; others arrive from the widely dispersed areas of the cortex by way of long or short *association fibers.* The corpus callosum *(commissural fibers)* links together corresponding regions of the two hemispheres. The maze of connections present within the cortex offers innumerable opportunities for circulation of nerve impulses; the mechanisms which preserve orderliness instead of chaos in these circuits are unknown.

The pattern of distribution of cortical cells varies in different regions of the brain. On the basis of such morphological characteristics — some obvious, others very subtle — several cytoarchitectural maps have been drawn up, parcelling the cerebrum into areas. Some areas have specialized functions, but for many no clear correspondence with function has been proved. The numbers by which Brod-

146

mann designated the anatomical areas in his chart, 52 in all, are still used frequently for descriptive purposes (Fig. 44).

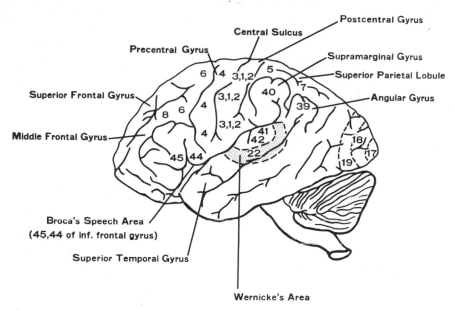

FIGURE 44. Lateral view of the brain depicting the most significant areas of Brodmann.

Motor Functions of the Cerebral Cortex

The *primary motor region* (area 4) is located in the *precentral gyrus* and rostral portion of the *paracentral lobule*. The largest neuronal cell bodies of the cerebral cortex, the Betz cells, are located in layer V of this region. They give rise to a very small percentage of the fibers in the corticospinal tract (CST). The other, smaller neurons in area 4 give rise to a significant portion of the CST. This area of the cortex controls fine, highly skilled, "voluntary" movements, particularly of the facial muscles and distal flexure musculature of the extremities. The facial region is represented on the ventrolateral aspect of the precentral gyrus (and gives rise, in part, to the corticobulbar tract); the leg is represented on the dorsomedial portion (see Fig. 43).

Lesions in the primary motor region give rise initially to flaccid paralysis of the contralateral musculature with hypotonia and decreased deep tendon reflexes. This is followed in a few weeks by remarkable recovery of function, the only deficits being a possible Babinski sign and decreased ability to perform skilled movements.

147

No spasticity results. In order to obtain spasticity and increased deep tendon reflexes, both the primary and supplementary motor areas must be involved.

A *supplementary motor area* is present on the medial surface of area 6 just rostral to the primary motor area. The parts of the body are represented in a somatotopic pattern which is somewhat reversed from that of the primary motor area in that the upper body components are located dorsal to those of the lower body. This region is apparently concerned with bilateral synergistic movements and unilateral lesions produce no permanent deficits.

The *premotor area* includes areas 6 and 8. Area 6 lies immediately in front of area 4 and continues on the medial surface to the cingulate gyrus. Area 6 is concerned with the development of motor skills and probably contains mechanisms for the elaboration of motor acts of more complex character than those represented in the motor area itself. This area also has subcortical connections with the coordination nuclei of the thalamus (the ventral anterior and ventral lateral nuclei) by which it is linked to the corpus striatum and to the cerebellum. Since these structures have motor functions but are not a part of the pyramidal system, they belong to the extrapyramidal systems. The premotor area is the cortical extrapyramidal center. Area 8 represents the frontal eye fields and is located in the caudal aspect of the middle frontal gyrus. Stimulation of this region causes conjugate deviation of the eyes to the opposite side.

Prefrontal Cortex

The large remaining part of the frontal lobe lying rostral to the motor and premotor areas is known as the *prefrontal region* and includes areas 9 through 12. Besides its connections with the dorsomedial nucleus of the thalamus, this part of the cerebral cortex receives an abundance of long association fibers from all other lobes. It is believed that this region is essential for abstract thinking, foresight, mature judgment, tactfulness, and forebearance. These regions do not, however, seem to be primarily concerned with intelligence as it is customarily tested.

The *symptoms* of patients with general paresis, whose frontal cortex is undergoing atrophy from syphilis, are chiefly mental. There is usually a lack of a sense of responsibility in personal affairs, slovenliness in personal habits, vulgarity in speech, and clownish behavior, frequently accompanied by feelings of euphoria. Similar symptoms may be encountered with tumors of the frontal lobe.

The operation of *prefrontal leukotomy* (or *lobotomy*) consists of severing the connections of the prefrontal area with the dorsomedial nucleus of the thalamus by driving a pick through the roof of the orbit and sweeping it across the fibers in a coronal plane. Identical effects have been produced by passing a needle into the dorsomedial nucleus and destroying it by cautery. The resulting changes in personality include a loss of anxiety and mental agitation. The disturbed psychotic patient becomes complacent and agreeable. These benefits are not achieved without undesirable changes in character. The patient is easily distracted, lacks initiative, shows poor judgment and lowered standards. The cortical scar that remains from the surgical lesion frequently causes epilepy.

PRIMARY SENSORY RECEPTIVE AREAS

Three primary receptive areas of the cortex contain the terminations of specific sensory nuclei of the thalamus. Fibers from the lateral geniculate body conveying visual impulses go to the cortex of the lips of the *calcarine fissure* (area 17). A lesion here produces contralateral hemianopia. Fibers from the medial geniculate body carry auditory impulses to the *anterior transverse gyrus* (Heschl), area 41. Unilateral lesions of this area have little effect because both ears have remaining connections to the intact temporal lobe. The ventral posterior nucleus relays tactile and proprioceptive impulses to the *postcentral gyrus*, the *primary somesthetic area* (areas 3, 2, and 1). Sensations of touch, pressure, and position are impaired on the opposite side of the body after lesions in this area, but pain and temperature sensations are not abolished. Similar to the primary motor cortex, the face is represented ventrolaterally on the postcentral gyrus, and the leg dorsomedially.

Before the arriving sensory messages are fully comprehended, they must undergo elaboration and analysis in an extensive cortical zone adjacent to the primary sensory area, the *sensory association area*.

Secondary Somesthetic Sensory Area

A *secondary somesthetic sensory area* exists which is located on the most ventral aspect of the pre- and postcentral gyri and extends caudally for a short distance along the superior lip of the lateral cerebral fissure. It is somatotopically organized such that the upper body components are represented rostral to those of the lower body. Although most of the body is represented contralaterally, some parts

149

have a bilateral input. This area receives input from several sensory modalities but pain predominates.

SENSORY ASSOCIATION AREAS

The *somesthetic* association area lies next to the postcentral gyrus in the parietal lobe (areas 5 and 7); the *visual* association area surrounds the visual area on the medial and lateral aspects of the occipital lobe (areas 18 and 19); and the *auditory* association area occupies a part of the superior temporal gyrus (areas 42 and 22) near the auditory area. The supramarginal (area 40) and angular (area 39) gyri are also important association areas which interrelate somesthetic, visual, and auditory stimuli. These associations have the tasks of formulating sensory stimuli into object images and of comprehending their meaning. This—the process of "knowing" or *gnosis*—must entail a comparison of present sensory phenomena with past experience. For example, the visual association areas must be called upon when an old friend is recognized in a crowd.

Lesions which are limited to the visual association areas (areas 18 and 19) do not cause blindness. Objects that are clearly seen but cannot be recognized and identified is a condition known as *visual agnosia*. Lesions of the parietal lobe (area 40) posterior to the somesthetic area produce tactile and proprioceptive agnosia. In addition to a loss of the ability to recognize familiar objects by feeling and handling them *(astereognosis)*, there is frequently a disturbance of body-image. One extremity may be ignored, or there may seem to be a phantom third limb. Individual fingers may not be recognized and the left and right sides of the body may be confused.

The auditory and visual association zones border upon an extensive, and relatively "silent," area of the temporal lobe in which visual and auditory sensory experience apparently are placed in storage as if they had been permanently recorded on sound film. It is here that the unknown mechanisms of memory, hallucinations, and dreams may be located. By stimulating an isolated point of the superior temporal gyrus in a conscious patient, Penfield has been able to evoke a detailed and vivid remembrance of a specific, but unimportant, event which had taken place several years previously. Epileptic seizures caused by focal irritation in the temporal lobe may be ushered in by hallucinations of sound. Occasionally they are preceded by memory disturbances in which present and past experiences are confused so that an event of the present seems to be a repetition of something that has happened before, the déjà vu phenomenon. Memory recording is temporarily suspended during a temporal lobe seizure. The patient may continue to carry out purposive movements, but he remains amnesic for the attack. A further indication of the importance of the temporal lobes in memory function is that removal of both lobes in humans permanently abolishes memory of past experiences.

Apraxia, Aphasia, Alexia, and Agraphia (Geschwind's Theory)

Apraxia is loss of the ability to carry out purposive, skilled acts, even though the sensory and motor systems are intact. The accomplishment of a voluntary action requires a larger part of the cortex than the motor and motor coordination systems alone. There must first be an idea—a mental formulation of the plan. This formula must then be transferred by association fibers to the motor system where it can be executed. Generalized cortical damage may cause apraxia by interfering with the general planning of voluntary acts. Lesions in the region of the supramarginal gyrus apparently cause apraxia by cutting off inpulses in association tracts. The idea is formed correctly but mistakes occur in translating it into performance. For example, when he is asked to drive a nail into a board, the patient may grasp the head of the hammer and strike the nail with the handle.

Facile use of language and speech is a remarkable attribute of the human brain—one that is shared by no other animal. A disturbance of language function as a result of brain injury concerns those forms of agnosia and apraxia which interfere with the use of written and spoken word symbols. This is known as *aphasia* (Fig. 45). Beginning early in life, nearly every individual trains one hemisphere of the brain more intensively than the other in the processes of association. It is usually the left side of the brain that assumes the leading role and the person becomes right handed. With rare exception, language function is also relegated to the hemisphere of motor dominance. *Aphasia does not appear unless a lesion is located in the dominant hemisphere.* If it becomes necessary, the speech centers of the nondominant hemisphere can be developed successfully in young, immature brains. Thus a right-handed child of five who suffers an injury in the left hemisphere will learn to speak perfectly again in a year or two. An adult may make this transfer but only after long intensive training, and even then the results may be imperfect.

1. *Lesion of Broca's area*

Broca's area is located in the caudal part of the inferior frontal gyrus (areas 44 and 45) immediately rostral to the motor area for the tongue, pharynx, and larynx. A lesion of this area in the *dominant hemisphere* causes *nonfluent, agrammatical*

151

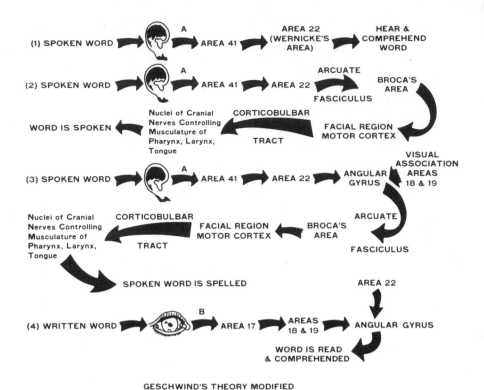

(1) SPOKEN WORD → A → AREA 41 → AREA 22 (WERNICKE'S AREA) → HEAR & COMPREHEND WORD

(2) SPOKEN WORD → A → AREA 41 → AREA 22 → ARCUATE FASCICULUS → BROCA'S AREA

WORD IS SPOKEN ← Nuclei of Cranial Nerves Controlling Musculature of Pharynx, Larynx, Tongue ← CORTICOBULBAR TRACT ← FACIAL REGION MOTOR CORTEX

(3) SPOKEN WORD → A → AREA 41 → AREA 22 → ANGULAR GYRUS → VISUAL ASSOCIATION AREAS 18 & 19

Nuclei of Cranial Nerves Controlling Musculature of Pharynx, Larynx, Tongue ← CORTICOBULBAR TRACT ← FACIAL REGION MOTOR CORTEX ← BROCA'S AREA ← ARCUATE FASCICULUS

SPOKEN WORD IS SPELLED

AREA 22

(4) WRITTEN WORD → B → AREA 17 → AREAS 18 & 19 → ANGULAR GYRUS

WORD IS READ & COMPREHENDED

GESCHWIND'S THEORY MODIFIED

FIGURE 45. Diagrammatic representation of the various association areas of the cerebrum related to language and writing comprehension.

aphasia (also referred to as expressive or motor aphasia). Without any paralysis of the lips, tongue, or vocal cords, the patient is unable to speak intelligibly. He knows what he intends to say, but cannot speak properly. The speech is very slow and many prepositions, nouns, and verbs are deleted. The patient has extreme difficulty in expressing certain grammatical words and phrases. "No ifs, ands, or buts" is a particularly difficult phrase to speak.

2. *Lesion of Wernicke's area*

Wernicke's area is located in the caudal aspect of the superior temporal gyrus (area 22). *Usually this area is larger on the dominant hemisphere than on the opposite side.* A lesion of this area in the dominant hemisphere causes *fluent, paragrammatical aphasia* (also referred to as auditory receptive or sensory aphasia). Voices are heard, but the words seem meaningless. The patient can speak, but makes many mistakes unknowingly because his failure in comprehension includes those words spoken by himself as well as by others. The patient speaks rapidly and without close inspection may sound normal (thus the term paragrammatical). His speech, however, lacks content and contains many meaningless (empty) words. Incorrect words are frequently substituted in the place of correct ones. Because of its interconnections with the angular gyrus (discussed below), and thus with visual association areas, damage to Wernicke's area results in difficulty comprehending both the spoken and written language.

3. *Lesion of the angular gyrus*

The angular gyrus (area 39) is the caudal part of the inferior parietal lobule located at the caudal aspect of the lateral cerebral fissure. It is situated between, and interconnected with, the supramarginal gyrus and Wernicke's area. The primary visual cortex (area 17) and the visual association areas (18 and 19) send fibers to this gyrus. A lesion of this area in the dominant hemisphere results in the loss of ability to read *(alexia)* and write *(agraphia)*. The patient can speak and understand spoken language as long as the arcuate fasciculus connection between Wernick's area and Broca's area is intact. Words can be seen but not comprehended.

As a result of its complex interconnections with auditory and visual association areas, the angular gyrus interrelates reading, writing, and speech. Normally, in order to understand a written word it must first be converted to the auditory form. On the other hand, in order to spell a spoken word, it must first be converted into the visual pattern. This explains why a patient with a lesion in this area can neither recognize words spelled aloud to him, nor spell aloud a spoken word.

4. *Lesion of the supramarginal gyrus*

The supramarginal gyrus (area 40) is the rostral part of the inferior parietal lobule. It interconnects with the primary and secondary somesthetic areas and with other association areas. Lesions in this region of the dominant hemisphere may possibly produce contralateral astereognosis.

5. *Conduction aphasia (disconnection syndrome)*

Broca's area, the supramarginal gyrus, the angular gyrus, and Wernicke's area are all cortical gray matter association regions which are interconnected by a subcortical bundle of association fibers, the *arcuate fasciculus*. If this fasciculus is interrupted, thus disconnecting Wernicke's area from Broca's area, *conduction aphasia* results. Speech is fluent but abnormal, and comprehension is intact. Repetition of spoken language is extremely difficult for the patient to achieve.

The Internal Capsule

Afferent and efferent fibers of all part of the cerebral cortex converge toward the brain stem forming the *corona radiata* deep in the medullary substance of the brain. When these fibers enter the diencephalon they become the *internal capsule*—a broad, compact band which separates the lenticular nucleus laterally from the caudate nucleus and thalamus medially. As seen in horizontal section, the internal capsule is shaped like a "V" with an *anterior* and a *posterior limb* joined at the *genu* (Fig. 46). Descending fibers of the pyramidal system are grouped closely at the genu and in the anterior two-thirds of the posterior limb. The corticomesencephalic and corticobulbar fibers for movements of the muscles of the head are located at the genu. Motor fibers of the upper extremity occupy the rostral part of the posterior limb and behind these are the lower extremity fibers. Fibers passing to and from the frontal lobe, other than pyramidal fibers, make up the anterior limb of the capsule, while those of the parietal lobe occupy the posterior part of the posterior limb. Optic and auditory radiation fibers are found in the sublenticular part of the internal capsule which is below the plane of section.

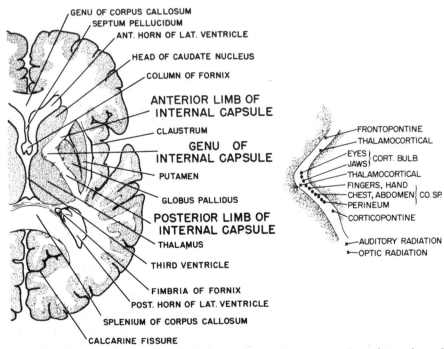

FIGURE 46. Horizontal section of the internal capsule showing the relationship of various tracts within the anterior limb, genu, and posterior limb.

154

THE CEREBRAL ARTERIES

The *middle cerebral artery,* a terminal branch of the internal carotid, enters the depth of the lateral fissure and divides into cortical branches which spread in a radiating fashion to supply the insula, and the lateral surface of the frontal, parietal, occipital and temporal lobes. The lenticulostriate arteries are small branches, variable in position and arrangement, which come from the basal part of the middle cerebral artery to supply the internal capsule and other nearby structures. In the presence of arteriosclerosis and high blood pressure, one of the branches may rupture and cause hemorrhage into the substance of the internal capsule. The sudden collapse which such an accident produces is commonly spoken of as a "stroke." A relatively small hemorrhage in this region results in widespread paralysis because all pyramidal tract fibers are contained in one small area. There is usually complete hemiplegia with signs of spasticity appearing after the initial period of shock. Sensory losses may also be produced if the fibers to the parietal lobe are included. Extensive hemorrhages are fatal, but after a less severe insult, the patient survives and may regain partial use of his limbs through restored function in some of the damaged nerve fibers.

An occlusion of the main trunk of the middle cerebral artery by the formation of a clot *(thrombosis)* produces paralysis of the opposite side of the body with preponderant effect in the face and upper extremity, hypesthesia in the same regions, partial hemianopia, and total aphasia (if located in the left hemisphere of a right-handed person). When individual cortical branches are occluded, the symptoms are limited to the loss of function in that particular region. For example, if the inferior frontal branch on the left is thrombosed, there is weakness of the lower part of the right face and tongue with motor aphasia.

The *anterior cerebral artery* turns medially to enter the median longitudinal cerebral fissure. On reaching the genu of the corpus callosum it curves dorsally and turns backward close to the body of the corpus callosum, supplying branches to the medial surface of the frontal and parietal lobes, and also to an adjoining strip of cortex along the top of the lateral surface of these lobes (Figs. 47 and 48). A small recurrent branch (medial striate), given off near the base of the artery, supplies the anterior limb and genu of the internal capsule. Thrombosis along the course of the anterior cerebral artery produces paresis and hypesthesia of the opposite lower extremity.

The basilar artery, a continuation of the fused vertebral arteries, bifurcates at the rostral border of the pons to form the posterior cerebral arteries. These arteries curve dorsally around the cerebral

155

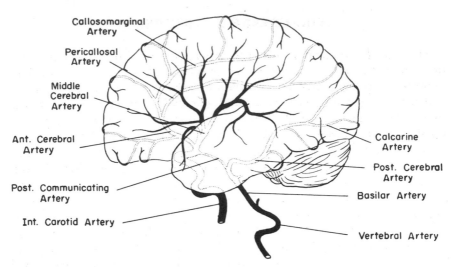

FIGURE 47. Left lateral view of the principal arteries of the cerebrum. The anterior cerebral and the posterior cerebral arteries, on the medial surface, are seen as if projected through the substance of the brain.

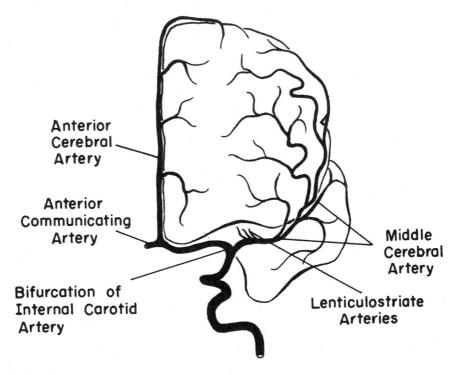

FIGURE 48. Anterior view of the anterior and middle cerebral arteries of the left hemisphere.

156

peduncles and send branches to the medial and inferior aspects of the temporal lobe, and to the occipital lobe (see Fig. 47). A separate branch, the calcarine artery, supplies the visual cortex. A number of perforating branches are given off which supply the posterior and lateral parts of the thalamus, and the subthalamus. Occlusion of the thalamic branches produces the thalamic syndrome. Sensations of touch, pain and temperature are distorted on the opposite side of the body. Superficial stimuli may produce disagreeable painful sensations, and agonizing, burning pain may occur spontaneously. In addition to the sensory changes, symptoms of cerebellar asynergia and tremor are produced in the extremities of the opposite side from damage to fibers of the superior cerebellar peduncle ascending to the ventral lateral nucleus of the thalamus. The calcarine branch of the posterior cerebral artery may be occluded independently of the thalamic branches. In this case the only sign produced will be contralateral hemianopia.

Circulus Arteriosus and Central Branches

The *circulus arteriosus* (circle of Willis) is formed by the junction of the basilar artery with the internal carotid arteries through the presence of a pair of posterior communicating arteries and an anterior communicating artery. (The communicating arteries are quite

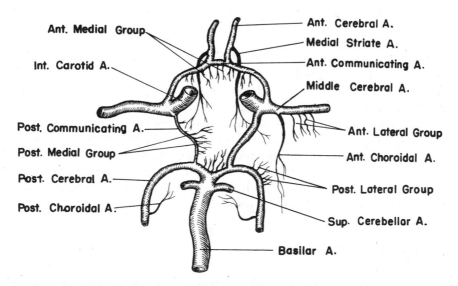

FIGURE 49. Diagram illustrating the origin of the central branches from the circulus arteriosus.

anomalous and the diagram purposely shows one posterior vessel somewhat smaller.) All the major cerebral vessels have their origin from the arterial circle (Fig. 49).

The central arteries supply the structures within the interior of the brain—the diencephalon, corpus striatum, and internal capsule. These vessels are branches of the arterial circle and may be conveniently considered in four groups:

Anterior medial group

Origin—anterior cerebral and anterior communicating arteries.

Distribution—anterior perforated substance to supply anterior hypothalamic region (preoptic and supraoptic regions).

Posterior medial group

Origin—posterior cerebral and posterior communicating arteries.

Distribution—posterior perforated substance.

Rostral group—tuber cinereum, stalk and hypophysis. Deeper branches penetrate thalamus.

Caudal group—mammillary bodies, subthalamus, and medial portions of thalamus and midbrain.

Anterior lateral group

Origin—primarily from the middle cerebral arteries; the *medial striate* or *anterior recurrent* from the anterior cerebral arteries.

Distribution—posterior perforated substance

Medial striate—anterior limb and genu of the internal capsule.

Lateral striate—basal ganglia and anterior limb of internal capsule.

These vessels are also known as lenticulostriate arteries.

Posterior lateral group

Origin—posterior cerebral artery.

Distribution—caudal portion of thalamus (geniculate bodies, pulvinar, and lateral nuclei).

Anterior and posterior choroidal arteries

These are considered to be central branches.

Anterior vessel arises from the middle cerebral arteries and supplies choroid plexus of lateral ventricles, hippocampus, some of the globus pallidus, and posterior limb of internal capsule.

Posterior choroidal artery arises from the posterior cerebral arteries and supplies the choriod plexus of the third ventricle and the dorsal surface of the thalamus.

Angiography

Angiography or arteriography refers to the procedure in which arteries of the brain (generally) are studied by x-ray following injection of the vessels with radiopaque material. The internal carotid or the vertebral arteries generally serve as the site of injection.

Cerebral angiography has been useful in determining the site of aneurysms and any anomalous development of the larger branches of the cerebral arterial circle. Edema or hemorrhage and tumors sometimes may be localized by the alteration in the arterial pattern.

Generally, the smaller terminal arteries are not identified by this procedure. Injection of the internal carotid artery outlines the anterior and middle cerebral arteries. The major branches of the basilar artery (cerebellars and posterior cerebral arteries) are outlined following injection of the vertebral artery. The posterior communicating artery, if it is sizable, might be apparent following either injection.

24

The Basal Ganglia and Related Structures

Motor activity is intricately controlled by the interaction of three major systems, the cerebral cortex, cerebellum, and basal ganglia. The cerebrum exerts its influence on the lower motor neurons either directly through the *pyramidal system* (cortiocospinal and cortico-bulbar tracts), or indirectly through polysynaptic, *extrapyramidal pathways* (for example, corticoreticulospinal tract and corticorubro-spinal tract; see Chapter 4). *Although technically incorrect, the term extrapyramidal system is restricted clinically to denote the components of the basal ganglia and related subcortical nuclei that influence motor activity.*

BASAL GANGLIA AND RELATED STRUCTURES

Aside from the fact that the interrelations of the basal ganglia are complex, the terminology used in describing these structures is quite confusing. *A thorough understanding of the terminology is an essential prerequisite for understanding the interconnections of this system.*

The major components of the basal ganglia include the *caudate nucleus,* the *putamen,* and the *globus pallidus.* Although some authorities include the amygdaloid nuclear complex and the claustrum, they will not be considered in this discussion. Two other subcortical nuclei, the *subthalamic nucleus* and the *substantia nigra,* are not specifically part of the basal ganglia per se, but are functionally very closely related. Table 2 should assist in learning the terminology associated with this system.

Table 2. Basal Ganglia Nomenclature

Term	Descriptive Terms Prefix	Descriptive Terms Suffix	Synonym	Components
Striatum	Strio-	-striate -striate	Neostriatum	Caudate and Putamen
Pallidum	Pallido-	-pallidal	Paleostriatum	Globus Pallidus
Lenticular Nucleus				Putamen and Globus Pallidus
Corpus Striatum				Caudate, Putamen, and Globus Pallidus
Subthalamic Nucleus	Subthalamo-	-subthalamic		
Substantia Nigra	Nigro-	-nigral		Pars compacta and Pars reticularis

After studying the chart, it should be apparent that "nigrostriatal" would be a proper name for a pathway that arises in the substantia nigra and terminates either in the putamen or caudate nucleus (or in both). Similarly, "pallidosubthalamic" would be an appropriate name for a pathway that arises in the globus pallidus and projects to the subthalamic nucleus. Notice that "corpus striatum" and "striatum" are not synonymous terms. They are frequently mistaken to be equivalent.

The *caudate nucleus* occupies a position in the floor of the lateral ventricle, dorsolateral to the thalamus (Fig. 50). The bulge at the cephalic end of the caudate is known as the *head*. The *body* passes backward at the side of the thalamus and tapers gradually to form the *tail* which curves ventrally and follows the inferior horn of the lateral ventricle into the temporal lobe ending near the amygdala. Some authorities subdivide the caudal nucleus into only a head and a tail.

The *lenticular*, or *lentiform nucleus* (see Fig. 50) is a thumb-sized mass wedged against the lateral side of the internal capsule. It is separated from the caudate nucleus by fibers of the internal capsule except in the cephalic part where these two nuclear masses fuse around the border of the anterior limb of the capsule. The lenticular nucleus is divided into the *putamen* and the *globus pallidas*. The putamen is the lateral portion having the same histological appearance as the caudate nucleus. The globus pallidus, in the same medial region of the lenticular nucleus, contains more large cells and is transversed by many myelinated fibers which accounts for its pale appearance in the fresh state.

The *subthalamus* (Fig. 51) is closely related to the basal ganglia in functions and contains the *zona incerta* (located between the lenticular fasciculus and the thalamic fasciculus), the *subthalamic reticular nucleus,* and the *subthalamic nucleus* (Luys). The zona incerta and

161

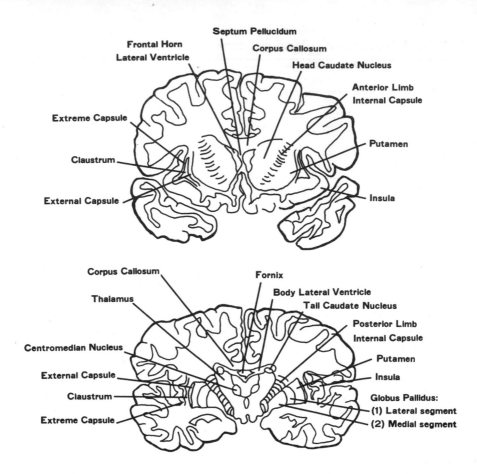

FIGURE 50. Frontal brain section depicting the components of the basal gangial at rostral (upper diagram) and caudal (lower diagram) levels.

the subthalamic reticular nucleus (the scattered cells in the prerubral field) are considered by some to be a rostral continuation of the midbrain reticular formation. The rostral portions of the *substantia nigra* and the *red nucleus* extend into the region. The subthalamic nucleus, lens-shaped and lying along the medial border of the internal capsule, is contiguous to the substantia nigra at its caudal extent.

Connections of the Basal Ganglia

The major outflow of efferent fibers from the basal ganglia comes from the globus pallidus (medial segment) (see Fig. 51). Some of

162

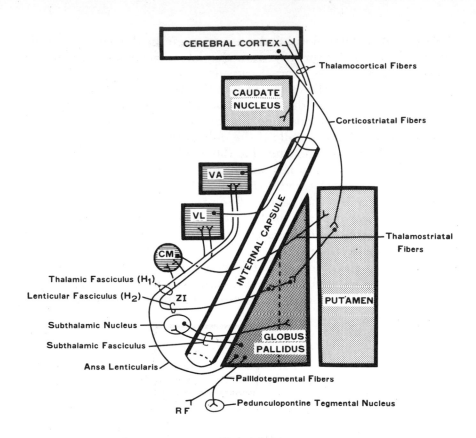

BASAL GANGLIA CONNECTIONS

FIGURE 51. Block diagram depicting many of the basal ganglia connections. CM = centromedian nucleus of the thalamus, RF = reticular formation of the brain stem, VA = ventral anterior nucleus of the thalamus, ZI = zona incerta of the ventral thalamus (subthalamic region).

these fibers stream directly across the posterior limb of the internal capsule. Upon entering the subthalamic region, they form a bundle which is known as the *lenticular fasciculus* (Forel's field H_2) located immediately ventral to the zona incerta (ZI). Another bundle of fibers from the globus pallidus (medial segment) passes around the ventral aspect of the posterior limb of the internal capsule to form a loop, the *ansa lenticularis.* Both bundles merge together on the medial aspect of the ZI in the *prerubral field* (Forel's field H) where they are joined by dentatothalamic fibers. The bundles then curve dorsally and pass laterally just dorsal to the ZI to form a discreet bundle which is called the *thalamic fasciculus* (Forel's field H_1). The fibers in these systems synapse in the *centromedian, ventral lateral,* and *ventral anterior* nuclei of the thalamus. A third bundle of

efferent fibers (pallidosubthalamic) arises from the globus pallidus (but in this case, primarily from the lateral segment), crosses the posterior limb of the internal capsule, and synapses in the subthalamic nucleus. Finally, a fourth bundle arises from globus pallidus (medial segment) and descends as *pallidotegmental fibers* to terminate in the pedunculopontine nucleus in the caudal aspect of the midbrain. The latter bundle is the only pathway that arises from the basal ganglia to descend caudal to the level of the substantia nigra.

The *substantia nigra* is a subcortical nucleus that is very closely related to the basal ganglia (Fig. 52). It is reciprocally connected with the striatum and sends efferents to the *ventral lateral* and *ventral anterior* thalamic nuclei. Neurons that arise in the pars compacta of the substantia nigra transmit dopamine, an inhibitory substance, to the striatum.

There are many circuits and feedback loops within and between the structures related to the basal ganglia. One very significant circuit is the following: cerebral cortex→ striatum→ globus pallidus→

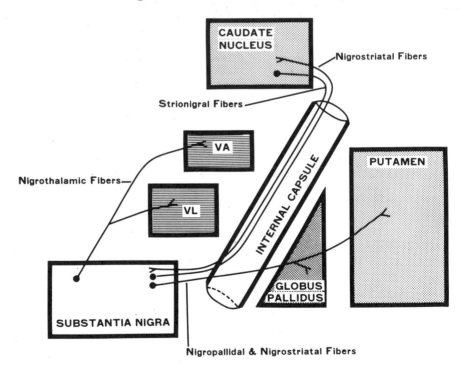

SUBSTANTIA NIGRA CONNECTIONS

FIGURE 52. Block diagram depicting the connections of the substantia nigra with other basal ganglia components and thalamic nuclei.

thalamus→ cerebral cortex. Another loop includes: cortex→ striatum→ substantia nigra→ thalamus→ cortex. Many smaller circuits exist between structures that have reciprocal connections (for example substantia nigra ⇌ striatum, and subthalamic nucleus ⇌ pallidum).

It is now possible to determine how the cerebral cortex, cerebellum, and basal ganglia interact. The cerebellum projects to the ventrolateral nucleus of the thalamus (through the dentatothalamic tract), which also receives projections from the pallidum and the substantia nigra. The ventrolateral nucleus projects to the primary motor region of the cerebral cortex. In turn, the motor cortex (and other regions of the cerebrum) projects to the striatum to enter the basal ganglia circuit, it then projects to the pons to enter the cerebellar circuit (corticopontocerebellar, Purkinje cells, dentate nucleus, and dentatothalamic tract). Consequently, both systems are constantly influencing part of the cerebral cortex that gives rise to the descending motor pathways (pyramidal and extrapyramidal) which effect the activity of the lower motor neurons.

Functional Considerations

Parkinson's disease, or paralysis agitans, is a common disease associated with degeneration in various parts of the basal ganglia and in the substantia nigra. The deep reflexes are usually normal, but muscle tonus is increased in a manner described as rigidity. Upon passively flexing or extending one of the extremities, an increased resistance is felt which gives way and returns in an alternating, jerky fashion like a cog-wheel. The rigidity of Parkinsonism affects all muscles without the special emphasis on the flexors of the upper extremity and the extensors of the lower extremity usually seen in diseases of the pyramidal system. In addition, there is tremor which is likely to be worse in a position of relaxation than when a voluntary movement is being carried out (resting tremor). Alternating movements of flexing and extending the fingers produce a characteristic "pill-rolling" tremor. The lines of the face are smooth, the expression fixed (masked face), and there is no spontaneous emotional response. The patient stands with head and shoulders stooped and walks with short, shuffling steps. The arms are held at the sides and do not swing in rhythm with the legs as they should, automatically. Although there is difficulty in starting to take the first steps, once under way the pace becomes more and more rapid, and the patient has trouble in stopping his progress when he reaches his goal. Parkinsonism patients show degenerate changes in the pallidum and substantia nigra (loss of and degeneration of neurons and an increase of glial cells). Destruction of the globus pallidus or the ansa lenticularis will stop the tremor on the opposite side of the body, and various surgical procedures to accomplish this aim have been attempted.

Chorea is also caused by damage to the basal ganglia, but instead of rigidity the chief manifestations are sudden, involuntary muscle movements. Choreiform movements are quick, jerky and purposeless. Facial grimaces may occur, or any part of the body may be affected. A vascular lesion in the basal ganglia may produce hemichorea involving only one side of the body. *Sydenham's chorea* occurs in children as a complication of rheumatic fever, but the damage is not permanent and recovery is complete. *Huntington's chorea* is an inherited disease with defects in the cerebral cortex as well as in the corpus striatum. This disease becomes progressively worse and leads to severe mental deterioration.

Athetosis is a form of striatal disease in which slow, writhing movements of a worm-like character appear in the extremities, chiefly in the fingers and wrists. Athetosis is frequently seen in association with spastic paralysis of the extremities in infants with brain damage which occurred at, or prior to birth.

Hemiballismus is an uncommon disease which is characterized by continued wild, flail-like movements of one arm. This is caused by a small lesion which damages the subthalamic nucleus on the opposite side.

25

The Cerebrospinal Fluid

The brain and spinal cord are suspended in cerebrospinal fluid, a clear watery liquid which fills the subarachnoid space surrounding them. The four ventricles of the brain are also filled with this fluid. The total quantity of fluid in adults is estimated to be 135 cc on the average. It is constantly being renewed by the production and reabsorption of some 400 to 500 cc of cerebrospinal fluid daily, a rate sufficient to replace it three times in 24 hours. Small amounts of protein, sugar, chlorides, and a very few lymphocytes (3 to 5 per cu mm) are present in the fluid. Its general composition is that of a blood ultrafiltrate passed through a semipermeable membrane with some modifications due to selective action.

Formation and Circulation of Cerebrospinal Fluid

Much of the fluid is formed in the *choroid plexuses* which are tufts of dilated capillaries that project into the walls of the ventricles in certain regions. There are two large plexuses in the floor of the lateral ventricles supplemented by smaller ones in the roofs of the third and fourth ventricles.

There is slow movement of fluid from the ventricles into the subarachnoid spaces from which it is absorbed by cerebral veins and removed by the blood stream. The fluid leaves the lateral ventricles through the *interventricular foramina,* traverses the third ventricle, and reaches the fourth ventricle by way of the *cerebral aqueduct*—the narrowest passageway of its entire route (Fig. 53). Three

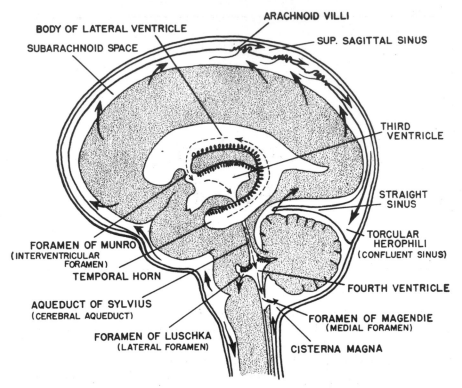

BODY OF LATERAL VENTRICLE

SUBARACHNOID SPACE

ARACHNOID VILLI

SUP. SAGITTAL SINUS

THIRD VENTRICLE

STRAIGHT SINUS

TORCULAR HEROPHILI (CONFLUENT SINUS)

FOURTH VENTRICLE

FORAMEN OF MUNRO (INTERVENTRICULAR FORAMEN)

TEMPORAL HORN

AQUEDUCT OF SYLVIUS (CEREBRAL AQUEDUCT)

FORAMEN OF LUSCHKA (LATERAL FORAMEN)

FORAMEN OF MAGENDIE (MEDIAL FORAMEN)

CISTERNA MAGNA

FIGURE 53. The circulation of the cerebrospinal fluid.

openings in the fourth ventricle allow the cerebrospinal fluid to pass from the internal channels into the subarachnoid space outside the brain. The two *lateral ventricular* apertures are located in the lateral recesses of the fourth ventricle; the *median ventricular aperture* is in the midline of the roof of the fourth ventricle. Small pockets of cerebrospinal fluid are found within the subarachnoid space in various locations around the base of the brain. The largest of these is the *cisterna magna* between the inferior surface of the cerebellum and the medulla. Other cisterns, the pontine, interpeduncular, and chiasmatic, lie between the base of the brain and the floor of the cranial cavity. The *cisterna superior (cisterna ambiens)* is the pocket of fluid which lies dorsal to the midbrain.

Spinal fluid fills the tubular extension of the subarachnoid space which forms a sleeve around the spinal cord. The lower limit of this space is variable, but on the average it is at the body of the second sacral vertebra, considerably below the end of the spinal cord. Although the spinal subarachnoid space is, in effect, a blind pocket, exchange of spinal fluid takes place by a slow mixing process induced by changes in posture.

Cerebrospinal fluid diffuses upward from the basal areas of the brain over the convexities of the hemispheres until it reaches the *arachnoid villi* in the walls of the superior sagittal sinus. It is absorbed from these villi and incorporated into the venous blood stream. Supplementary routes for reabsorption of cerebrospinal fluid have been proposed, but it is questionable whether these are very effective. A small amount may be absorbed from the spinal space by the vessels of the sheaths of emerging nerves. The veins and capillaries of the pia mater may also be capable of removing some cerebrospinal fluid.

The *Virchow-Robin* spaces are funnel-like extensions from the subarachnoid space which surround the walls of blood vessels as they enter the substance of the brain. For many years it was believed that these perivascular spaces were filled with cerebrospinal fluid and that they continued around the capillaries to connect with small fluid spaces around neurons. On the basis of studies made with the electron microscope it has been concluded that the Virchow-Robin spaces do not extend beyond arterioles.

The Pressure of the Cerebrospinal Fluid

Any obstruction to the normal passage of cerebrospinal fluid causes the fluid to back up in the ventricles and leads to a general increase of intracranial pressure. After the pressure has been elevated for some time, usually a matter of days or weeks, the effect can be seen by inspecting the fundus of the eye with an ophthalmoscope. Due to the high pressure inside the sleeve of dura mater which surrounds the optic nerve, the retinal veins are dilated and the optic nerve head (optic disc) is pushed forward above the level of the retina. This is known as *papilledema*, or *choked disc*. If papilledema has persisted for a long time, the fibers of the optic nerve will be damaged and the disc assumes a chalk-white color instead of the normal pale pink.

The most common cause of papilledema is a tumor of the brain compressing some part of the ventricular system. Tumors far removed from the ventricles may not produce obstruction until they reach very large size. A tumor of the cerebellum generally exerts pressure on the roof of the fourth ventricle, and, since it is confined within the posterior fossa by the semi-rigid tentorium cerebelli with little room for expansion, it is likely to cause early obstruction to the flow of cerebrospinal fluid through the fourth ventricle. Tumors near the orbital surface of one frontal lobe may compress the optic nerve and produce optic atrophy in that eye, while the other eye develops papilledema from generalized elevation of pressure as the tumor expands in size, the Foster Kennedy syndrome. Other cardinal signs of brain tumor in addition to papilledema are persistent headache and vomiting. The headache is probably caused from the stretching of nerve endings in the dura mater. Irritation of the vagal nuclei in the floor of the fourth ventricle accounts for nausea and vomiting.

Hydrocephalus is an excessive accumulation of cerebrospinal fluid. Fluid sometimes collects in the subarachnoid space over the external surface of the brain following meningitis or trauma, but most cases of hydrocephalus are the result of blockage along the passage-ways and the extra fluid is in the ventricles of the brain. In *congenital hydrocephalus* an open path for cerebrospinal fluid fails to develop normally. Other developmental anomalies are also likely to be present. The head usually appears to be of normal size at birth, but it begins to show a disproportionate enlargement during the first few months. The thin skull, with its widely open sutures, offers little resistance to pressure from within and gradually swells to enormous proportions. Meanwhile the ventricles become greatly dilated and the brain substance is reduced to a thin shell. Obstructions of the cerebral aqueduct by an overgrowth of ependymal cells may prevent the passage of fluid from the third to the fourth ventricle, or a malformation of the medial and lateral apertures may block the out-flow from the fourth ventricle. Frequently the stoppage is caused by an elongation of the medulla and cerebellum downward into the foramen magnum. This permits fluid to escape into the space around the spinal cord, but it cannot ascend to the basal cisterns above the foramen magnum. In such cases a dye injected into one of the lateral ventricles can be recovered by needle puncture of the subarachnoid space in the lumbar region and the condition is known as *communicating hydrocephalus.*

Samples of cerebrospinal fluid for diagnostic tests are obtained by directing a long needle between two upper lumbar vertebrae and inserting it far enough to reach and pierce the dura mater. There is no danger of injuring the nerve roots of the cauda equina which are present at this level. With the patient relaxed and in a recumbent position the pressure of the spinal fluid should not exceed 150 mm of H_2O. The pressure rises to about 300 mm H_2O with the patient in the sitting position. Small oscillations of the fluid level in a manometer connected to the needle arise from the transmission of the cerebral pulse. These pulsations indicate that free communication is present. If blockage of the spinal subarachnoid space is suspected, the *Queckenstedt test* can be performed. With the needle in place and a water manometer attached, the jugular veins are compressed for ten seconds. Under normal conditions there will be a rapid rise and fall in pressure, normal levels returning within 15 seconds. This is a negative test. The test is positive if no change in pressure occurs. The test should never be performed if symptoms of elevated intracranial pressure are present because of the danger of cerebellar tonsil herniation. Even lumbar punctures should be performed cautiously in the presence of elevated intracranial pressure, since the release of pressure from below may allow similar herniation. If the medulla protruded into the foramen magnum, death could result from damage to the cardiac and respiratory centers.

Spinal fluid can also be obtained by passing a needle at the base of the skull directly through the atlanto-occipital membrane into the cisterna magna. No nervous structures are encountered, but the needle would strike the medulla if it should slip too far and, for this reason, cisternal puncture is not often attempted by inexperienced persons.

Pneumoencephalography

If the pineal body is calcified, its shadow may be seen in x-rays and displacement in its position may give significant information. Thinning or erosion of skull bones, as shown by x-ray, may help to establish the presence of a mass in the adjacent parts of the brain. Most tumors, however, cannot be visualized directly unless they are partly calcified. If the cerebrospinal fluid is completely withdrawn from the ventricular spaces and replaced by air, these spaces will appear as shadows in an x-ray. Dilations, distortions in shape, and filling defects can then be studied in considerable detail. This process—*pneumoencephalography*—is accomplished by means of lumbar puncture. If the intracranial pressure is increased, lumbar puncture cannot be performed safely and it is necessary to introduce air directly into the ventricular system to obtain a visible outline by x-ray—*ventriculography.* This process requires the drilling of trephine holes in the parietal bones through which needles can be passed into both lateral ventricles.

Index

ABDOMINAL reflexes, loss of, 43
Abducens nerve, 56, 79
   functional components of, 67
   nucleus of, 58
Accessory cuneate nucleus, 32
Accessory nerve, 51, 69, 70
Accommodation, 117
Acoustic nerve, 56, 86
Acoustic stria
   dorsal, 87
   intermediate, 87
   ventral, 88
Acupuncture anesthesia, 27
Adiadochokinesia, 104
Adie's pupil, 117
Adrenal gland, sympathetic innervation
   of, 123
Adrenergic nervous system, 121
Afferent, 10
Afferent fibers, 2
   of cranial nerves, 63
   of spinal nerves, 10
Afferent pathways of cerebellum, 100-102
Agnosia, visual, 150
Agraphia, 153
Alexia, 153
Allocortex, 145
Alpha motor neurons, 9, 13-14
Alternating hemiplegia, 105
Amyotrophic lateral sclerosis, 44-45
Analgesia, alternating, 84
Angiography, 158-159
Angular gryus, lesion of, 153
Anosmia, 143
Ansa lenticularis, 163

Anterior corticospinal tract, 21
Anterior funiculus, 6
Anterior horns, 6
   lesions of, 44
   pyramidal tracts and, lesions of, 44-45
Anterior lobe of cerebellum, 98
Anterior median fissure, 6
Anterior medullary velum, 56
Anterior spinal artery, thrombosis of, 45
Anterior spinothalamic tract, 36-37
   effect of cutting of, 38
Anterior transverse temporal gyrus, 89
Anterior white commissure, 25
Anterolateral system, 24-30, 36-37
   in hemisection of spinal cord, 46
Aphasia, 151-153
   conduction, 153
Apraxia, 151
Arachnoid villi, 169
Archicerebellum, 97-98
Archicortex, 145
Arcuate fasciculus, 153
Argyll Robertson pupil, 117
Artery(ies)
   anterior spinal, 45
   cerebral, 155-159
Astereognosis, 34, 35, 150
Asthenia, 104
Asynergia, 100
Ataxia, 35, 103
Athetosis, 166
Atrophy of muscles, 40
Auditory pathway, 87-89
Auditory reflexes, 90
Auditory system, 86-90

Autonomic fibers, 3
Autonomic nervous system, 120-126
Axon, 1

BABINSKI'S sign, 41, 42
Basal ganglia, 127
  connections of, 162-163
  dysfunctions of, 165-166
  nomenclature of, 161
  related structures and , 160-166
Basilar membrane of ear, 86-87
Basilar portion of pons, 56
Bell's palsy, 81
Benedikt's syndrome, 110-111
Bipolar olfactory epithelial cells, 66
Bladder
  atonic, 126
  automatic, 126
  innervation of, 124-126
  sympathetic supply to, 124
Body temperature, regulation of, 131
Bony spiral lamina, 86
Brachium, 2
Brachium conjunctivum, 100
Brachium pontis, 100
Brain, 2
Brain stem, 5, 50-62. See also Medulla;
    Pons; Midbrain.
  cranial nerve nuclei in, anatomical po-
      sition of, 64-65
  lesions of, 105-111
Broca's area, lesion of, 151-152
Brodmann's area 4, 18
Brown-Séquard syndrome, 45-46
Bulbar accessory nerve, 73

CALAMUS scriptorius, 51
Calcarine fissure, 114, 149
Cardiac muscles, 3
Cardiac nerves, 122
Carotid body reflex, 77
Carotid plexus, 122
Carotid sinus reflex, 76
Cauda equina, 6
Caudate nucleus, 160, 161
Cells, nerve, 1-2
Cell body, 1
Central gray matter, 52
  lesions of, 44
Central nervous system, 3-9
Central sulcus of Rolando, 3
Central tegmental tract, 57-58
Cerebellar ataxia, 100
Cerebellum, 97-104
  afferent pathways of, 100-103
  cortex of, 98-99
  dysfunction of, signs of, 103-104
  efferent pathways of, 100-103

feed-back circuits through, 102-103
  hemispheres of, 97
  lobes of, 98
  nuclei of, 58
  peduncles of. See Peduncles, cere-
      bellar.
  subdivisions of, 97-100
  synergistic function of, 100-103
Cerebral aqueduct, 59, 167
Cerebral arteries, 155-159
Cerebral cortex
  arteries of, 155-159
  Brodmann's areas, 146-147
  motor areas of, 18
    descending fibers from, 20-23
  motor functions of, 147-148
  neurons of, 145-149
  prefrontal, 148-149
  sensory association areas of, 150-154
  sensory receptive areas of, 149-150
Cerebral peduncles, 56, 60
Cerebrospinal fluid
  diagnostic tests on, 170-171
  formation and circulation of, 167-169
  pressure of, 169-171
Cerebro-olivocerebellar system, 101
Cerebroreticulocerebellar system, 101
Cerebrum, 3-5
Cervical ganglia, 122
Cervical sympathetic trunk, 122
Choked disc, 169
Cholinergic nervous system, 121
Chorea, 166
Choroid plexus, 50, 167
  of third ventricle, 127
Chromatolysis, 48
Chromophilic substance, 48
Ciliary ganglion, 116
Ciliospinal reflex, 119
Circle of Willis, 157
Circulus arteriosus, 157
Cisterna ambiens, 168
Cisterna magna, 168
Cisterna superior, 168
Clarke's nucleus, 6
Clasp-knife response, 41
Clava, 51
Clonus, 41
Cochlea, 86
Cochlear nerve, 87
Cochlear nuclei, 87
Colliculus (i)
  inferior, 60, 61, 88
  superior, 60, 61
Column, 2
Commissural, 9
  fibers, 146
Conjugate eye movements, 93, 94

173

Conus medullaris, 6
Consensual light reflex, 116
Convergence, 117
Corneal reflex, 84-85
Corona radiata, 154
Corpora quadrigemina, 60
Corpus callosum, 3
Corticobulbar tract, 21
Corticomammillary pathway, 129
Corticopontine tracts, 58, 101
Corticopontocerebellar pathways, 101
Corticoreticulospinal system, 22
Corticorubrospinal system, 22
Corticospinal tract, 20-21, 42, 54. *See also* Pyramidal tract.
Corticotectal tract, 21-22
Cough reflex, 77
Cranial nerves. *See also* Nerves.
    functional components of, 63-69
    of medulla, 70-78
    of pons and midbrains, 79-85
Cranial outflow, 121
Cremasteric reflex, loss of, 43
Crossed extension reflexes, 16-17
Crus cerebri, 59, 60, 61
Cuneate tubercle, 51
Cuneocerebellar tract, 32
Cuneus, 115

DEAFNESS. *See* Hearing, defects of.
Decerebrate rigidity, 93
Decomposition of movement, 103
Decussation of Forel, 61
Decussation of pyramidal tract, 21
Deep cerebellar nuclei, 97
Déjà vu phenomenon, 150
Dendrites, 1
Dentate nucleus, 97
Denticulate ligaments, 6
Dermatome, 28
Descending motor pathways, 18-23
Diabetes insipidus, 130
Diencephalon, 5, 127-133
Diplopia, 79
Disconnection syndrome, 153
Dorsal arcuate fibers, 32
Dorsal column nuclei, 34
Dorsal column pathways, 34
Dorsal longitudinal fasciculus, 129
Dorsal roots, 6
    dorsal root zones and, of spinal cord, 31-35
    in hemisection of spinal cord, 46
    irritation of, sensory effects of, 28
    lesions of, 43
Double vision, 79
Dorsal nucleus of Clarke, 6

Dura mater, 6
Dural sac, 6
Dysdiadochokinesia, 103
Dysmetria, 103

EARS
    bilateral representation of, in temporal lobes, 89
Edinger-Wesphal nucleus, 116
Efferent, 10
Efferent fibers, 2
    of cranial nerves, 64
    of spinal nerves, 10
Efferent pathways of cerebellum, 100-103
Eighth nerve, *See* Acoustic nerve.
Eleventh nerve, *See* Accessory nerve.
Emboliform nucleus, 97
Endolymph, 87
Epithalamus, 140
Extrafusal muscle fibers, 14, 15
Extrapyramidal pathways, 160
Extrapyramidal system, 23, 160
Eye movements, 119

FACIAL colliculus, 52
Facial nerve, 56, 81-83
    functional components of, 67
    motor nucleus of, 58
Fasciculation of muscle, 40
Fasciculus, 2
    cuneatus, 34, 36, 54
    gracilis, 34, 36, 38, 54
    mammillaris princeps, 129
    medial longitudinal, 23, 55, 57, 61, 62, 94
    posterolateral, 24
    proprius, 17
Fastigial nucleus, 97
Fastigiobulbar tract, 92
Feed-back circuits through cerebellum, 102-103
Fibers
    afferent, 2, 10, 63
    autonomic, 3
    commissural, 146
    efferent, 2, 10, 64
    extrafusal muscle, 14, 15
    dorsal arcuate, 32
    internal arcuate, 54
    intrafusal muscle, 15
    motor, 3
    nerve. *See* Nerve fibers
    nuclear bag intrafusal, 15
    nuclear chain, 15
    pain, 24, 26
    peripheral autonomic, 1
    postganglionic, 1

projection, 146
proprioceptive, 31-34
sensory, 3
somatic, 3, 10
thalamocortical, 25-26, 38
Fibrillation of muscle, 40
Fifth nerve. See Trigeminal nerve.
Filum terminale, 6
Fissures, 3
anterior median, 6
calcarine, 114, 149
medial longitudinal, 3
of Sylvius, lateral, 3
Flexor reflexes, 16-17
Flocculonodular lobe, 97-98
Folia, 97
Fornix, 132
Fountain decussation of Meynert, 61
Fourth nerve. See Trochlear nerve.
Fourth ventricle, 50
Frontal lobe, 3
Functional components of spinal nerves,
10-12
Funiculus
anterior, 6
lateral, lesions involving, 45
posterior, 34, 38
in hemisection of spinal cord, 46
lesions involving, 45
signs of injury to, 35
Furrows, 3

GAG reflex, 77
Gait, posture and, distrubances of, 103
Gamma motor neuons, 9, 13-14
in spasticity, 41-42
Gamma system, reticular system and, 22
Ganglion(a), 1
basal. See Basal ganglia.
cervical, 122
hypogastric, 122
inferior mesenteric, 122
prevertebral, 122
spinal, 31
spiral, 87
terminal, 123
General visceral efferent fibers, 120
Geniculate bodies, 113
Geniculocalcarine tract, 113
Geschwind's theory, 151-153
Glands, 3
Globose nucleus, 97
Globus pallidus, 160, 161, 162
Glossopharyngeal nerve, 51, 75-76
branches of, 71-72
functional components of, 68
Gnosis, 150
Golgi tendon organs, 16

Granular layer of cerebellar cortex, 98-99
Gray matter, 1
Gray rami communicantes, 121
Gyrus, 3
angular, lesion of, 153
anterior transverse temporal, 89, 149
cingulate, 145
dentate, 145
of Heschl, 89, 149
parahippocampal, 145
postcentral, 34, 149
supramarginal, 153

HABENULAR commissure, 140
Habenular nuclei, 140
Habenulopeduncular tract, 140
Hearing, 86-90
defect of, 96
from nerve damage and mechanical
obstruction, 89
Hemianopia
heteronomous bitemporal, 115
homonymous, 114
Hemiballismus, 166
Hemiplegia, 42
alternating, 105
Hippocampus, 132, 145
Hoffmann's sign, 42
Horner's syndrome, 122
Huntington's chorea, 166
Hydrocephalus, 170
Hyperesthesia, 28
Hypnosis, 27
Hypogastric ganglia, 122
Hypoglossal nerve, 50, 70
functional components of, 69
nucleus of, 54
Hypoglossal trigone, 51
Hypophyseal portal system, 130
Hypothalamo-hypophyseal tracts, 129
Hypothalamic sulcus, 127
Hypotonia, 104
Hypothalamus, 127
appetite and centers of, 131
body temperature and, 131
emotion and, 131-133
fiber connections to, 128-129
limbic system and, 127-133
nuclei of, 128, 131
pituitary relationships to, 130

INCUS ossicle, 86
Inferior cerebellar peduncle, 51, 54,
99-100
Inferior mesenteric ganglia, 122
Infundibulum, 128
Intermediolateral cell column, 22
Intermediolateral gray columns, 6, 9

Internal arcuate fibers, 54
Internal capsule, 127, 154
  lesion of, 40-41
Internal medullary lamina, 134
Internal strabismus, 79
Interneurons, 13
Internode, 2
Internuncial cells, 13
Interpeduncular fossa, 59
Intersegmental reflexes, 13
Interstitiospinal tract, 23, 55, 57
Interthalamic adhesion, 127
Interventricular foramen, 127, 167
Intrafusal muscle fibers, 15
Isocortex, 145

JUXTARESTIFORM body, 92

KINESTHETIC sense. See Proprioception.

LAMINAE of Rexed, 9
Lateral cervical system, 36-37, 39
Lateral corticospinal tract, 21
Lateral fissure of Sylvius, 3
Lateral funiculi, 6
Lateral lemniscus, 61, 87., 89
Lateral reticulospinal tract, 22
Lateral spinothalamic tract, 38
  effect of cutting of, 27-28
Lateral ventricles, 168
Lemniscus, 2
Lenticular fasciculus, 163
Lenticular nucleus, 161
Lentiform nucleus, 161
Lesion(s)
  angular gyrus, 153
  anterior horns and pyramidal tracts,
    44-45
  brain stem, 105-111
  Broca's area, 151-152
  central gray matter, 44
  corticospinal tract, 42
  internal capsule, 40-41
  lower motor neuronal, 19, 40, 42
  medulla, 105-107
  midbrain, 110-111
  motor pathway, 42-43
  of motor region, 147
  of nerves and spinal cord, 40-49
  of pons, 107-110
  of posterior roots, 43
  of visual pathway, 114-115
  of Wernicke's area, 152-153
  peripheral nerve, 43
  pontocerebellar angle, 109
  supramarginal gyrus, 153
  upper motor neuronal, 19, 40-42, 80-82
Leukotomy, prefrontal, 148

Light reflex, 116
Limbic lobe, 133
Limb position, inability to recognize, 35
Lingual gyrus, 115
Lissauer's tract, 24
Lobes, 3
Lobotomy, 148
Lower motor neurons, 20
  in proprioception pathways, 32
  lesions of, 19, 40, 42
Lumbar splanchnic nerves, 122

MALLEUS ossicle, 86
Mammillary bodies, 127, 128
Mammillary nuclei, 132
Mammillotegmental fasciculus, 129
Mammillothalamic tract, 132
Massa intermedia, 127
Mastication muscles, 83
Medial eminence, 52
Medial forebrain bundle, 129
Medial geniculate body, 62, 88
Medial lemniscus, 34, 57, 61
  decussation of, 54
Medial longitudinal fasciculus, 23, 55, 57,
    61, 62, 94
Medial longitudinal fissure, 3
Medial reticulospinal tract, 22, 23
Medial vestibulospinal tract, 55
Medulla, 5, 50-55
  cranial nerves of, 70-78
  external markings of, 50-52
  internal structures of, 52-55
  lesions of
    basal part of, 105-106
    central region of upper, 106-107
    dorsolateral region of, 107
Medullary reticulospinal tract, 22
Ménière's syndrome, 96
Mesocortex, 145-146
Midbrain, 5, 59-62
  cranial nerves of, 79-85
  external markings of, 59-60
  internal structures of, 60-62
  lesions of
    basal part of, 110
    superior colliculi of, 111
    tegmentum of, 110-111
Middle cerebellar peduncle, 56, 57, 100
Millard-Gubler's syndrome, 108
Mimetic muscles, 81
Molecular layer of cerebellar cortex,
    98-99
Monoplegia, 42
Monosynaptic reflex arc, 13
Motion sickness, 96
Motor areas of cerebral cortex, 18-23
Motor fibers, 3

Motor neurons, 20
Motor pathways
  descending, 18-23
  lesions of, reflexes associated with,
    42-43
Multiple neuritis, 43
Muscle(s)
  atrophy of, 40
  cardiac, 3
  mastication, 83
  mimetic, 81
  movement of, 13
  paralysis of. *See* Paralysis.
  skeletal, 3
  smooth, 3
  spasticity of, 41-42
  spindles, 14-15
  synergy, 100
  tone, 13-17
  tonus, 15
Mydriasis, 80
Myelin sheath, 1
Myotatic reflex, 16

NEGATIVE feedback, 14
Neocerebellum, 98
Neocortex, 145-146
Nerve(s)
  abducens. *See* Abducens nerve.
  accessory. *See* Accessory nerve.
  acoustic, 56·
  cardiac, 122
  cranial. *See* Cranial nerves.
  facial. *See* Facial nerve.
  glossopharyngeal. *See* Glosso-
    pharyngeal nerve.
  hypoglossal. *See* Hypoglossal nerve.
  oculomotor, 60, 66, 80-81
  olfactory, 66
  optic, 66
  spinal. *See* Spinal nerves.
  spinal cord and, lesions of, 40-49
  trigeminal. *See* Trigeminal nerve.
  trochlear. *See* Trochlear nerve.
  vagus. *See* Vagus nerve; Vagal system.
  vestibular, 91-93
  vestibulocohlear, 67-68
Nerve cells, 1-2
  degenerative changes in, 47-48
Nerve fibers, 1-2
  bundles of, terms for, 2
  classification of, 11-12
  designation of, 10-11
  regeneration of, 49
Nervus intermedius, 71, 75
Neurolemma, 1
Neurolemma cells, 49
Neuron(s), 1, 2

  alpha motor, 9, 13-14
  gamma motor, 9, 13-14
    in spasticity, 41-42
  lower motor, 20
  upper motor, 20
Neuropile, 2
Neurotransmitter, 2
Ninth nerve. *See* Glossopharyngeal
    nerve.
Nissl substance, 48
Nodes of Ranvier, 2
Nuclear bag intrafusal fiber, 15
Nuclear chain fiber, 15
Nucleus (i), 1
  ambiguus, 55
  dentatus, 58
  dorsal column, 34
  dorsalis, 6, 9, 32
  emboliformis, 58
  fastigii, 58, 92
  globosus, 58
  of Bechterew, 91
  of Deiter, 91
  of Schwalbe, 91
  ventral posterolateral, 34
Nystagmus, 104
  vestibular, 94-95

OBEX, 50
Occipital lobe, 3
Oculomotor nerve, 60, 80-81
  functional components of, 66
Olfactohypothalamic pathway, 129
Olfactory apparatus, peripheral, 141-142
Olfactory bulbs and striae, 141-142
Olfactory cortex, 145
Olfactory epithelium, 141
Olfactory nerve, 66
Olfactory reflexes, 142-144
Olivary nuclear complex, 51
  inferior, 54
Olive, 51
  superior, 57
Optic chiasm, 112, 127
Optic chiasma, 127
Optic nerve, 112, 113
  functional components in, 66
Optic radiation, 113
Optic reflexes, 116-119
Optic tracts, 113
Organ of Corti, 87, 89
Ossicles of middle ear, 86

PAIN
  gate-controlled mechanism and, 27
  perception of, 26-27
  radicular, 28
  receptors, 24

reflexes, 30, 119
  temperature sensibility and, 27-30
  visceral and referred, 28-30
Pain-temperature pathways, 24-30
Paleocerebellum, 98
Paleocortex, 145
Pallidotegmental fibers, 164
Papilledema, 169
Paracentral lobule, 147
Parahippocampal gyrus, 133
Paralysis
  agitans, 165
  cerebral arteries and, 155
  facial, 81-83
  flaccid, 40
  of left lateral gaze, 110
  of right lateral gaze, 108
  of upward gaze, 111
  spastic, 40-42
Paraplegia, 42, 93
Parasthesia, 28
Parasympathetic nervous system
  cranial division of, 124
  urinary bladder and, 124-126
Paravertebral ganglion, 121
Paresis, 42, 148
Parietal lobe, 3
Parinaud's syndrome, 111
Parkinson's disease, 165
Pathway(s)
  auditory, 87-89
  descending motor, 18-23
  dorsal column, 34
  of proprioception. See Proprioceptive
    pathways.
  of simple touch, 36-39
  pain-temperature, 24-30
  posterior column, 34
  spinal cord, 36
  spinocervicothalamic, 36, 39
Peduncle(s), 2
  cerebellar
    inferior, 51, 54, 99-100
    middle, 56, 57, 100
    superior, 56, 59, 100
      decussation of, 61
  cerebral, 56, 60
Perikaryon, 1
Peripheral autonomic fibers, 1
Peripheral nerves, lesions of, 43
Peripheral nervous system, 2-3
Pia mater, 6
Pineal body, 127, 140
Pneumoencephalography, 171
Poliomyelitis, acute, 44
Pons, 5
  basilar portion of, 56
  cranial nerves of, 79-85

external markings of, 56
internal structure of, 56-59
lesions of
  basal caudal part of, 107-108
  middle region of, 109-110
Pontine nuclei, 57
Pontine reticulospinal tract, 22, 23, 55, 57
Pontocerebellar angle, 56
  lesions of, 109
Postcentral gyrus, 34
Posterior funiculus. See Funiculus, pos-
    terior.
Posterior gray horns, 6
Posterior lobe of cerebellum, 98
Posterior median sulcus, 6
Posterior nerve roots. See Dorsal nerve
    roots.
Postsynaptic neuron, 2
Posterolateral fasciculus, 24
Postganglionic fibers, 1
Postganglionic neuron, 120
Posture, gait and, disturbances of, 103
Precentral gyrus, 147
Preganglionic neuron, 120
Preganglionic parasympathetic cell
    bodies, 11
Preganglionic sympathetic cell bodies, 11
Premotor cortex, 18
Prerubral field, 163
Presynaptic neuron, 2
Pretectal area, 116
Prevertebral gangila, 122
Primary motor area, 18
Projection fibers, 146
Proprioception and stereognosis, 31-35
Proprioceptive fibers, 31-34
Proprioceptive pathways
  directly upward in posterior funic-
    ulus, 34
  interruption of, disturbances following,
    35
  to lower motor neurons, 32
  to spinocerebellar pathways, 32-33
Propriospinal system, 17
Protective reflexes, 16, 118
Ptosis, 80, 122
Pupil, Argyll Robertson, 117
Pupillary constriction, 117
Purkinje cell layer of cerebellar cortex,
    98-99
Putamen, 160, 161
Pyramids, 50, 56
Pyramidal tract, 20-21, 160
  anterior horns and, lesions of,
    44-45
  decussation of, 21
  in hemisection of spinal cord, 46
  syndrome, classical, 41

Quadriplegia, 42
Queckenstedt test, 170

Recurrent collaterals, 14
Red nucleus, 61, 162
Reflex(es)
    abdominal, 43
    associated with near-point reaction,
        117
    auditory, 90
    carotid body, 77
    carotid sinus, 76
    ciliospinal, 119
    corneal, 84-85
    cough, 77
    cremasteric, 43
    flexor and crossed extension, 16-17
    gag, 77
    in lesions of motor pathway, 42-43
    intersegmental, 13
    light, 116
    myotatic, 16
    olfactory, 141-144
    optic, 116-119
    pain, 30, 119
    protective, 16, 118
    salivary-taste, 76
    spinal, 13-17
    stretch, 15-17
    vagal system, 76-78
    visual fixation, 117-118
    vomiting, 78
Renshaw cell, 14
Restiform body, 99. See also Peduncle,
    cerebellar, inferior.
Reticular formation, 25-26, 52
Retina, 113
Rhinencephalon and olfactory reflexes,
    141-144
Rinné test, 90
Romberg sign, 35, 43
Round window, 87
Rubrospinal tract, 61

Saccule, 91-92
Salivatory nucleus, 74
Salivary-taste reflex, 76
Saltatory conduction, 2
Scala tympani, 86-87
Scala vestibuli, 86-87
Scanning speech, 104
Schwann cells, 49
Scotoma, 114
Second nerve. See Optic nerve.
Secondary motor area, 18
Secondary somatic sensory area, 26
Secondary somatosensory cortex, 18
Segmental reflexes, 13

Semicircular canals, 91
Sensory association areas, 150-154
Sensory dissociation, 44
Sensory fibers, 3
Sensory receptive areas, 149-150
Seventh nerve. See Facial nerve.
Sheath of Schwamm, 1
Simple reflex, 13
Simple touch, pathways of, 36-39
Sixth nerve. See Abducens nerve.
Skeletal muscle, 3
Smooth muscles, 3
Solitary tract, 55
Somatic, 10
Somatic afferent fibers, 10, 63
Somatic efferent fibers, 10, 64
Somatic motor fibers, 3
Somesthetic sensory area, 149-150
Spinal cord, 5-9
    dorsal roots and dorsal root zones of,
        31-35
    hemisection of, 45-56
    influence of descending pathways on,
        23
    lesions of, 40-49
    principal tracts of, 48
    tumors of, 46-47
Spinal ganglia, 31
Spinal nerves, 2, 6
    accessory, functional components of,
        69
    functional components of, 10-12
    lesions of, 40-49
Spinal reflexes, 13-17
Spinal tract of V, 26
Spindles, muscle, 14-15
Spinocerebellar tract, 32, 34
Spinocervical tract, 39
Spinocervicothalamic pathway, 36, 39
Spinothalamic tracts, 24
Spiral ganglion, 87
Squint, 79
Stapes ossicle, 86
Statoacoustic nerve, 67
Stereognosis, 31-34
Strabismus, external, 80
Stretch reflex, 15-17, 40-41
Striae medullares, 56, 140
Stria terminales, 129, 134
Stroke, 155
Subarachnoid space, 6
Substantia gelatinosa, 9
Substantia nigra, 60, 61, 160, 162, 164
Subthalamic nucleus, 160, 161-162
Subthalamic reticular nucleus, 161-162
Subthalamus, 161-162
Sulcus (i), 3
    limitans, 52

179

posterior median, 6
Superior cerebellar peduncle, 56, 59, 61, 100
Superior olivary nuclei, 88-89
Superior olive, 90
Supplementary motor area, 18
Supramarginal gyrus, lesion of, 153
Supraspinal reflexes, 13
Sydenham's chorea, 166
Sympathetic nervous system, 121-123
Sympathetic trunks, 121
Sympathectomy, 123
Synapse, 2
Synaptic cleft, 2
Synaptic vesicles, 2
Syndrome
    Benedikt's, 110-111
    Brown- Séquard, 45-46
    Horner's, 122
    Millard-Gubler's, 108
    of Foville, 108
    Parinaud's, 111
    posterior inferior cerebellar artery, 107
    Weber's, 110
Syringomyelia, 44
System(s)
    anterolateral, 24-30
    auditory, 86-90
    autonomic nervous, 120-126
    central nervous, 3-9
    corticoreticulospinal, 22, 41
    corticorubrospinal, 22, 41
    corticospinal, 20-21
    extrapyramidal, 23
    lateral cervical, 36-37, 39
    peripheral nervous, 2-3
    propriospinal, 17
    pyramidal, 20-21
    sympathetic nervous, 121-123
    vagal. See Vagal system.
    ventrolateral. See Anterolateral system.
    vestibular, 91-96

TABES dorsalis, 43
Tactile discrimination, 34, 36
Tactile senses, 36-39
Tectobulbar tract, 57
Tectospinal tract, 23, 55, 57, 61, 90
Tectum, 60, 90
    of midbrain, 60
Tegmental decussation, 61
Tegmentum, 56, 60
Temperature sense, 27-30
Temporal lobe, 3
    bilateral representation of ears in, 89
Tenth nerve, See Vagus nerve.
Tentorium cerebelli, 97
Terminal ganglia, 123

Terminal sulcus, 134
Thalamic fasciculus, 163
Thalamic nuclei, 25-27
Thalamocortical fibers, 25-26
Thalamus, 134-140
    nucleus of, 163-164
        connections of, 136-139
        functional categorization of, 139
    perception of pain and, 26-27
Third nerve. See Oculomotor nerve.
Thoracic splanchnic nerves, 122
Thoracolumbar outflow, 121
Tic douloureux, 85
Tinnitus, 89, 96
Tract(s), 2
    anterior spinothalamic, 36-37, 38
    central tegmental, 57-58
    corticobulbar, 21
    cortico-olivary, 58
    corticopontine, 58, 101
    corticospinal. See Corticospinal tract.
    corticotectal, 21-22
    cuneocerebellar, 32
    fastigiobulbar, 92
    hypothalamo-hypophyseal, 129
    interstitiospinal, 23, 55, 57
    lateral spinothalamic, 27-28, 38
    Lissauer's, 24
    of Russell, 92
    pyramidal, 20-21
    reticulospinal, 22, 23
        pontine, 22, 23, 55, 57
    rubro-olivary, 58
    rubrospinal, 61
    spinal, of V, 26
    spinocerebellar, 32, 34
    spinocervical, 39
    spinothalamic, 24
    tectobulbar, 57
    tectospinal, 23, 55, 57, 61, 90
    trigeminothalamic, 26, 84
    vestibulospinal, 23, 93
        medial, 55
Tractotomy, 27-28
Trapezoid body, 57
    nuclei of, 88-89
Tremor, 104
Trigeminal hemiplegia, alternating, 109
Trigeminal lemniscus, 84
Trigeminal nerve, 26, 56
    functional components of, 66
    motor division of, 83
    principal sensory nuclus of, 59
    sensory division of, 83-85
Trigeminal neuralgia, 85
Trigeminothalamic tract, 26, 84
Trochlear nerves, 60, 79
    functional components of, 66

nucleus of, 61
Tuber cinereum, 127
Tumor of brain, 169-170
Twelfth nerve. *See* Hypoglossal nerve.
Two point discrimination, loss of, 35
Tympanic membrane, 86

UPPER motor neurons, 20
  lesions of, 40-42
Urinary bladder. *See* Bladder.
Utriculus, 91

VAGAL system
  course and distribution of nerves of,
      71-73
  motor portion of, 73
  parasympathetic portion of, 73-75
  reflexes of, 76-78
  sensory portion of, 75-76
Vagal trigone, 51
Vagus nerve, 51, 72. *See also* Vagal sys-
      tem.
  branches of, 72-73
  dorsal motor nucleus of, 54, 73-75
  functional components of, 68
Vena terminalis, 134
Vermis, 97
Vertigo, 95-96
Ventral nerve roots, 6 '
  in hemisection of spinal cord, 46
Ventral posterolateral nucleus, 34
Ventriculography, 171
Ventrolateral system. *See* Anterolateral
  system.

Vestibular efferent fibers, 93
Vestibular group, nuclei of, 58
Vestibular nerve, 91-93
Vestibular nuclei, 91
  inferior, 55
Vestibular nystagmus, 94-95
Vestibular system, 91-96
Vestibulocochlear nerve, functional com-
      ponents of, 67-68
Vestibulo-ocular pathways, 93-94
Vestibulospinal tracts, 23, 93
Vibratory sense, loss of, 35
Virchow-Robin spaces, 169
Visceral, 10
Visceral afferent fibers, 10, 63, 64
Visceral efferent fibers, 10, 64
Vision, 112-115
Visual fields, 114
Visual fixation reflex, 117-118
Visual pathway, 112-115
  lesions of, 114-115
Visual receptive area, 114
Vomiting reflex, 78
Von Frey hairs, 38

WEBER test, 90
Weber's syndrome, 110
Wernicke's area, lesion of, 152-153
White matter, 1
White rami communicantes, 121

ZONA incerta, 161-162

181